The Language of Nursing Theory and Metatheory

Imogene M. King
Jacqueline Fawcett
Editors

Sigma Theta Tau International
Honor Society of Nursing

Center Nursing Press
550 West North Street
Indianapolis, Indiana 46202

Sigma Theta Tau International
Peer-reviewed Publications

Date	Title
1992	Leonard Felix Fuld, 19th Century Reformer in a 20th Century World
1997	The Image Editors: Mind, Spirit, and Voice
1997	The Language of Nursing Theory and Metatheory
1997	The Adventurous Years: Leaders in Action, 1973-1993, a Nell Watts memoir
1997	Virginia Avenel Henderson: Signature for Nursing
1998	The Neuman Systems Model and Nursing Education: Teaching Strategies and Outcomes
1998	Immigrant Women and Their Health: An Olive Paper
1999	The Communication of Caring in Nursing
1999	Roy Adaptation Model-Based Research: 25 Years of Contributions to Nursing Science
2000	Nurses' Moral Practice: Investing and Discounting Self

For other Center Nursing Press publications and videos, contact:
Sigma Theta Tau International
550 West North Street
Indianapolis, IN 46202
1.888.634.7575
FAX: 317.634.8188
nursingsociety.org/publication

Library of Congress Catalog Number: 96-072339
ISBN: 0-9656391-0-X

Printed in the United States of America

Views expressed herein
are not necessarily those of
Sigma Theta Tau International.

Table of Contents

Contributors

Jacqueline Fawcett, PhD, FAAN
Professor
University of Pennsylvania
School of Nursing
Philadelphia, PA

Joyce J. Fitzpatrick, PhD, FAAN
Elizabeth Brooks Ford Professor and Dean of Nursing
Case Western Reserve University
Frances Payne Bolton School of Nursing
Cleveland, OH

Hesook Suzie Kim, PhD, RN
Professor
University of Rhode Island
College of Nursing
Kingston, RI
Professor II
University of Oslo
Faculty of Medicine, Institute of Nursing Science

Imogene M. King, EdD, FAAN
Professor Emeritus
University of South Florida
College of Nursing
Tampa, FL

Maeona K. Kramer, PhD, RN
Professor of Nursing
University of Utah
College of Nursing
Salt Lake City, UT

Afaf Ibrahim Meleis, PhD, DrPS(hon), FAAN
Professor
University of California, San Francisco
School of Nursing
Department of Community Health Systems
San Francisco, CA

Patricia Munhall, PhD, FAAN
Professor
Barry University
College of Nursing
Miami, FL

Rosemarie Rizzo Parse, PhD, FAAN
Professor and Niehoff Chair
Loyola University
Marcella Niehoff School of Nursing
Chicago, IL

Mary Cipriano Silva, PhD, FAAN
Professor
Director, Center for Health Care Ethics
George Mason University
College of Nursing and Health Science
Fairfax, VA

Prologue

Imogene M. King
Jacqueline Fawcett

Every discipline passes through phases of change in the discovery of knowledge. As the discipline of nursing prepares to take its place at the center of the health care systems of the 21st century, it is imperative to review the past and present and offer ideas for the future of knowledge development. This monograph represents one way to review what has been, what is, and what might be in nursing knowledge development.

The discipline of nursing can take pride in its accomplishments with regard to theory development and the recognition of the relationship between research and theory development during the last few decades of the 20th century. Ample evidence documents the contributions that theory-based research has made to nursing practice, education, and administration. As we approach the dawn of a new century, it seems appropriate to reflect on the language of nursing theory and metatheory because that language ultimately is reflected in the language of the practical endeavors of research, practice, education, and administration.

This monograph is, as the title denotes, about the language of nursing theory and metatheory. As used in the title, nursing theory and metatheory are broad terms meant to connote the range of nursing knowledge. More specifically, nursing theory is meant to connote formal nursing knowledge that has been developed through reflection, along with philosophical, historical, and empirical inquiry. Metatheory refers to the nature of theory in general, or more specifically, knowledge about the nature and structure of the products of reflection and inquiry.

The terminology used to describe the components of nursing theory and metatheory varies widely. Most frequently, different terms are used to refer to the same level or component of nursing knowledge. For example, abstract frames of reference are variously labeled as conceptual models, conceptual frameworks, conceptual systems, theoretical frameworks, grand theories, theories, and paradigms. In addition, the same term may be used to refer to different components of nursing knowledge. The term, paradigm, for example, frequently is used to denote a philosophical position, a conceptual model, or an approach to research. The lack of consistency in terminology has created problems for students, faculty, and clinicians who are attempting to understand and appreciate formal nursing knowledge.

The impetus for this monograph was our concern about the confusion created by the diversity in terminology used to describe nursing knowledge, that is, nursing theory and metatheory. Although we did not think that we would be able to identify a common language, it was our intent to make explicit the terms used by major nursing scholars and their definitions of those terms. To that end, we invited several nurse scholars who are renowned for their work in nursing theory and metatheory to contribute to the monograph. We are especially gratified by the enthusiasm with which

Joyce Fitzpatrick, Hesook Suzie Kim, Maeona Kramer, Afaf Meleis, Patricia Munhall, Rosemarie Parse, and Mary Silva accepted our invitation.

This monograph, then, presents several short essays by nurse scholars about the terminology used for nursing knowledge. Each contributor was asked to identify the terms that she uses for nursing theory and metatheory, her definition for each term, and her philosophic and/or pragmatic rationale for the terminology. Chapters 1 through 9 present the essays authored by the invited nurse scholars as well as our own somewhat diverse ideas about the language of nursing theory and metatheory. Each of these nine chapters of the monograph presents its author's thinking about formal nursing knowledge.

We are grateful to Sigma Theta Tau International for the opportunity to publish this monograph. Although we anticipate that graduate students in courses dealing with nursing knowledge development will find the contents of this monograph especially helpful, the monograph was written for all nurse educators, researchers, and administrators; undergraduate, master's, and doctoral students; and clinicians. We hope that all readers will be excited and challenged by the ideas presented here and will accept our invitation to contribute their own ideas about the language of nursing theory and metatheory to the literature.

Chapter 1
The Structural Hierarchy of Nursing Knowledge: Components and Their Definitions
Jacqueline Fawcett

My ongoing analysis of contemporary nursing knowledge, viewed through the lens of my philosophic orientation to knowledge development, has led to the identification of five components that form a structural hierarchy. The five components and their levels of abstraction are depicted in **Figure 1**.

Philosophic Orientation

Prior to defining and describing each component of the structural hierarchy of contemporary nursing knowledge, I will share the basic tenets of my philosophy of knowledge development. I would like to first point out that I did not invent the labels used in what I have come to think of as the structural hierarchy of contemporary nursing knowledge; rather, I tried to make sense of and organize the labels found in the literature, with an emphasis on the development of empirical nursing knowledge.

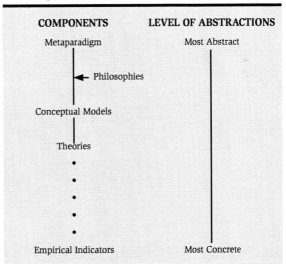

Figure 1: The structural hierarchy of contemporary nursing knowledge: Components and levels of abstraction.

My philosophic orientation is grounded in the belief that nursing is, as Donaldson and Crowley (1978) claimed, a professional discipline that encompasses basic, applied, and clinical research. Thus, I believe that all nursing knowledge is ultimately developed for the purpose of understanding what happens in the encounter between a nurse and a recipient of nursing. This belief has led me to adopt an empiricist orientation to knowledge development.

My version of empiricism is rooted in the postpositivistic position that all knowledge is developed within a conceptual and sociohistorical perspective (Lavee & Dollahite, 1991), and that all observation—in both research and clinical situations—is "theory-laden." More specifically, I believe, as Popper (1965) maintained, that all observations are made within a "frame of reference, [an] horizon of expectations" (p. 47), and that "Observation is always selective. It needs a chosen task object, a definite task, an interest, a point of view, a problem" (Popper, 1965, p. 46).

Moreover, I believe that there is a reciprocal relationship between the frame of reference and the observations. In particular, I believe that one cannot observe the world without observing it through some conceptual or theoretical frame of reference; the observations, in turn, can affect the frame of reference (Fawcett, 1992; Kahn & Fawcett, 1995). Ultimately, then, I believe that it is impossible to make "objective" observations, because all observations are made within the context of some conceptual model or theory.

Finally, I fully endorse Popper's (1965) stance that the goal of research is to refute or falsify hypotheses. Scientific progress is, I believe, hindered by a hypothesis that cannot be falsified because it cannot be modified or replaced by another hypothesis. Conversely, a falsifiable hypothesis can be improved or replaced by a better one. The aim, then, is to develop and empirically test falsifiable hypotheses that bring us successively closer to a comprehensive understanding of the nurse-recipient encounter.

The Components of the
Structural Hierarchy of Nursing Knowledge

The Metaparadigm

The first component of the structural hierarchy of contemporary nursing knowledge is the metaparadigm. Following Kuhn (1977), I have defined the metaparadigm of any discipline as the global concepts that identify the phenomena of interest to that discipline and the global propositions that state the relationships among those phenomena. I regard the metaparadigm as the most abstract component in the structural hierarchy of contemporary nursing knowledge, and as "an encapsulating unit, or framework, within which the more restricted ... structures develop" (Eckberg & Hill, 1979, p. 927).

Moreover, I view the metaparadigm as "the broadest consensus within a discipline, [which] provides the general parameters of the field and gives scientists a broad orientation from which to work" (Hardy, 1978, p. 38). The functions of a metaparadigm are to summarize the intellectual and social missions of a discipline and place a boundary on the subject matter of that discipline (Kim, 1989).

The phenomena of interest to nursing are, in my reasoned opinion, represented by four central concepts: person, environment, health, and nursing. Person refers to the recipient of nursing, including individuals, families, communities, and other groups. Environment refers to the person's significant others and physical surroundings, as well as to the setting in which nursing occurs, which ranges from the person's home to clinical agencies to society as a whole. Health is the person's state of well-being, which can range from high-level wellness to terminal illness. Nursing refers to the definition of nursing, the actions taken by nurses on behalf of or in conjunction with the person, and the goals or outcomes of nursing actions.

Nursing actions typically are viewed as a systematic process of assessment, labeling, planning, intervention, and evaluation.

The relationships among the metaparadigm concepts are described in four propositions (Donaldson & Crowley, 1978; Gortner, 1980). The first proposition links the person and health; it states that the discipline of nursing is concerned with the principles and laws that govern the life-process, well-being, and optimal functioning of human beings, sick or well.

The second proposition emphasizes the interaction between the person and the environment; it states that the discipline of nursing is concerned with the patterning of human behavior in interaction with the environment in normal life events and critical life situations.

The third proposition links health and nursing; it declares that the discipline of nursing is concerned with the nursing actions or processes by which positive changes in health status are effected.

The fourth proposition links the person, the environment, and health; it asserts that the discipline of nursing is concerned with the wholeness or health of human beings, recognizing that they are in continuous interaction with their environments.

Philosophies

The philosophy is the second component in the structural hierarchy of contemporary nursing knowledge. A philosophy may be defined as a statement of beliefs and values (Kim, 1989; Seaver & Cartwright, 1977). More specifically, philosophies are statements about what people assume to be true in relation to the phenomena of interest to a discipline (Christensen & Kenney, 1990), and what they believe regarding the development of knowledge about those phenomena. An example of a philosophic statement is "The individual...behaves purposefully, not in a sequence of cause and effect" (Roy, 1988, p. 32).

Philosophies of nursing encompass ethical claims about what nurses should do, ontological claims about the nature of human beings and the goal of nursing, and epistemic claims dealing with how nursing knowledge is developed (Salsberry, 1994). Ethical claims about nursing are summarized in the dominant collective philosophy of humanism (Gortner, 1990), which emphasizes "humanistic (moral) values of caring and the promotion of individual welfare and rights" (Fry, 1981, p. 5). Ontological and epistemic claims about nursing are summarized in three contrasting world views: reaction, reciprocal interaction, and simultaneous action (Fawcett, 1993, 1995).

Conceptual Models

The third component of the structural hierarchy is the conceptual model. The term conceptual model is synonymous with the terms paradigm, conceptual framework, conceptual system, and disciplinary matrix. A conceptual model is defined as a set of abstract and general concepts and the propositions that integrate those concepts into a meaningful configuration (Lippitt, 1973; Nye & Berardo, 1981).

A conceptual model provides a distinctive frame of reference—an "horizon of expectations" (Popper, 1965, p. 47)—and "a coherent, internally unified way of thinking about ... events and processes" (Frank, 1968, p. 45). Thus, a conceptual model tells its adherents how to observe and interpret the phenomena of interest to the discipline. Each conceptual model, then, presents a unique focus that has a profound influence on our perceptions of the world.

The works of several nurse scholars currently are recognized as conceptual models. Among the best known are *Johnson's Behavioral System Model*, *King's General Systems Framework*, *Levine's Conservation Model*, *Neuman's Systems Model*, *Orem's Self-Care Framework*, *Rogers' Science of Unitary Human Beings*, and *Roy's Adaptation Model* (Johnson, 1980, 1990; King, 1971, 1990; Levine, 1969, 1991; Neuman, 1995; Neuman & Young, 1972; Orem, 1971, 1995; Rogers, 1970, 1990; Roy, 1976; Roy & Andrews, 1991).

Theories

The next component in the structural hierarchy of nursing knowledge is the theory. A theory is less abstract than its parent conceptual model but more abstract than the empirical indicators that operationalize the theory concepts. Theories are made up of relatively specific and concrete concepts and propositions that purport to account for or organize some phenomenon (Barnum, 1994).

Theories vary in scope; that is, they vary in the relative level of concreteness and specificity of their concepts and propositions. Theories that are broadest in scope are called grand theories. These theories are made up of rather abstract and general concepts and propositions that cannot be generated or tested empirically. Indeed, grand theories are developed through thoughtful and insightful appraisal of existing ideas or creative intellectual leaps beyond existing knowledge. Examples of grand theories in nursing include Leininger's (1991) *Theory of Culture Care Diversity and Universality,* Newman's (1986, 1994) *Theory of Health as Expanding Consciousness,* and Parse's (1981, 1992) *Theory of Human Becoming.*

Middle-range theories are narrower in scope than grand theories, encompassing a limited number of concepts and a limited aspect of the real world. By definition, middle-range theories are made up of concepts and propositions that are empirically measurable. Examples of middle-range theories in nursing include Orlando's (1961) *Theory of the Deliberative Nursing Process,* Peplau's (1952, 1992) *Theory of Interpersonal Relations,* and Watson's (1985) *Theory of Human Caring.*

Empirical Indicators

The generation and testing of middle-range theories is accomplished through the use of empirical indicators, which are the fifth and final component in the structural hierarchy of contemporary nursing knowledge. Empirical indicators are the very specific and concrete real world proxies for middle-range theory concepts. More specifically, they are the actual instruments, experimental conditions, and research procedures that are used to observe or measure the concepts of a middle-range theory. For example, the *Relationship Form* (Forchuk & Brown, 1989) is the instrument that serves as the empirical indicator for the concept of the nurse-patient relationship in Peplau's (1952) *Theory of Interpersonal Relations*. This instrument measures the progress of the nurse-patient relationship through the four phases delineated by Peplau: orientation, identification, exploitation, and resolution.

Conclusion

The version of contemporary nursing that I have presented in this chapter has emphasized empirical knowledge. Such knowledge encompasses discursively written descriptions, explanations, or predictions of objective or subjective phenomena that are based on group data and are capable of being publicly refuted (Carper, 1978). Empirical knowledge is frequently equated with scientific theory.

I do, however, recognize the need for and value of ethical, personal, and esthetic knowledge, as those forms of knowledge have been defined by Carper (1978) and Chinn and Kramer (1995). Ethical knowledge, which is discursively written as standards, codes, and normative ethical theories, emphasizes the values of nurses and nursing. Such knowledge focuses on the value of changes and outcomes in terms of desired ends, and it addresses questions of moral obligation, moral value, and nonmoral value. Personal knowledge is expressed as the authentic and disclosed self; it is not written or codified discursively. Personal knowledge is concerned with the knowing, encountering, and actualizing of the self, and with the wholeness and integrity in personal encounters between nurses and patients. It specifically addresses the quality and authenticity of the interpersonal process between each nurse and each patient. Esthetic knowledge, which is expressed as the art-act of nursing, addresses manual and technical skills as well as the nurse's perception of what is significant in the individual patient's behavior. This kind of knowledge focuses on the particulars of each individual rather than the universals of groups.

In summary, contemporary nursing knowledge is, in my view, a structural hierarchy that ranges from the global concepts and propositions of the metaparadigm to the concrete operations and instruments that permit empirical testing of concepts and propositions.

References

Barnum, B.J.S. (1994). **Nursing theory: Analysis, application, evaluation** (4th ed.). Philadelphia: J.B. Lippincott.

Carper, B.A. (1978). Fundamental patterns of knowing in nursing. **Advances in Nursing Science, 1(1),** 13-23.

Chinn, P.L., & Kramer, M.K. (1995). **Theory and nursing: A systematic approach** (4th ed.). St. Louis: Mosby-Year Book.

Christensen, P.J., & Kenney, J.W. (Eds.). (1990). **Nursing process: Application of conceptual models** (3rd ed.). St. Louis: C.V. Mosby.

Donaldson, S.K., & Crowley, D.M. (1978). The discipline of nursing. **Nursing Outlook, 26,** 113-120.

Eckberg, D.L., & Hill, L., Jr. (1979). The paradigm concept and sociology: A critical review. **American Sociological Review, 44,** 925-937.

Fawcett, J. (1992). Conceptual models and nursing practice: The reciprocal relationship. **Journal of Advanced Nursing, 17,** 224-228.

Fawcett, J. (1993). From a plethora of paradigms to parsimony in worldviews. **Nursing Science Quarterly, 6,** 56-58.

Fawcett, J. (1995). **Analysis and evaluation of conceptual models of nursing** (3rd ed.). Philadelphia: F.A. Davis.

Forchuk, C., & Brown, B. (1989). Establishing a nurse-client relationship. **Journal of Psychosocial Nursing and Mental Health Services, 27(2),** 30-34.

Frank, L.K. (1968). Science as a communication process. **Main Currents in Modern Thought, 25,** 45-50.

Fry, S. (1981). Accountability in research: The relationship of scientific and humanistic values. **Advances in Nursing Science, 4(1),** 1-13

Gortner, S.R. (1980). Nursing science in transition. **Nursing Research, 29,** 180-183.

Gortner, S.R. (1990). Nursing values and science: Toward a science philosophy. **Image: Journal of Nursing Scholarship, 22,** 101-105.

Hardy, M.E. (1978). Perspectives on nursing theory. **Advances in Nursing Science, 1(1),** 37-48.

Johnson, D.E. (1980). The behavioral system model for nursing. In J.P. Riehl & C. Roy, **Conceptual models for nursing practice** (2nd ed., pp. 207-216). New York: Appleton-Century-Crofts.

Johnson, D.E. (1990). The behavioral system model for nursing. In M.E. Parker (Ed.), **Nursing theories in practice** (pp. 23-32). New York: National League for Nursing.

Kahn, S., & Fawcett, J. (1995). Continuing the dialogue: A response to Draper's critique of Fawcett's "Conceptual models and nursing practice: The reciprocal relationship." **Journal of Advanced Nursing, 22,** 188-192.

Kim, H.S. (1989). Theoretical thinking in nursing: Problems and prospects. **Recent Advances in Nursing, 24,** 106-122.

King, I.M. (1971). **Toward a theory for nursing: General concepts of human behavior.** New York: John Wiley & Sons.

King, I.M. (1990). King's conceptual framework and theory of goal attainment. In M.E. Parker (Ed.), **Nursing theories in practice** (pp. 73-84). New York: National League for Nursing.

Kuhn, T.S. (1977). Second thoughts on paradigms. In F. Suppe (Ed.), **The structure of scientific theories** (2nd ed., pp. 459-517). Chicago: University of Illinois Press.

Lavee, Y., & Dollahite, D.C. (1991). The linkage between theory and research in family science. **Journal of Marriage and the Family, 53,** 361-373.

Leininger, M.M. (1991). The theory of culture care diversity and universality. In M.M. Leininger (Ed.), **Culture care diversity and universality: A theory of nursing** (pp. 5-65). New York: National League for Nursing.

Levine, M.E. (1969). **Introduction to clinical nursing.** Philadelphia: F.A. Davis.

Levine, M.E. (1991). The conservation principles: A model for health. In K.M. Schaefer & J.B. Pond (Eds.), **Levine's conservation model: A framework for nursing practice** (pp. 1-11). Philadelphia: F.A. Davis.

Lippitt, G.L. (1973). **Visualizing change. Model building and the change process.** Fairfax, VA: NTL Learning Resources.

Neuman, B. (1995). **The Neuman systems model** (3rd ed.). Norwalk, CT: Appleton & Lange.

Neuman, B., & Young, R.J. (1972). A model for teaching total person approach to patient problems. **Nursing Research, 21,** 264-269.

Newman, M.A. (1986). **Health as expanding consciousness.** St. Louis: C.V. Mosby.

Newman, M.A. (1994). **Health as expanding consciousness** (2nd ed.). New York: National League for Nursing.

Nye, F.I., & Berardo, F.N. (Eds.). (1981). **Emerging conceptual frameworks in family analysis.** New York: Praeder.

Orem, D.E. (1971). **Nursing: Concepts of practice.** New York: McGraw-Hill.

Orem, D.E. (1995). **Nursing: Concepts of practice** (5th ed.). St. Louis: Mosby Year Book.

Orlando, I.J. (1961). **The dynamic nurse-patient relationship**. New York: G.P. Putnam's Sons.

Parse, R.R. (1981). **Man-living-health: A theory of nursing**. New York: John Wiley & Sons.

Parse, R.R. (1992). Human becoming: Parse's theory of nursing. **Nursing Science Quarterly, 5,** 35-42.

Peplau, H.E. (1952). **Interpersonal relations in nursing**. New York: G.P. Putnam's Sons.

Peplau, H.E. (1992). Interpersonal relations: A theoretical framework for application in nursing practice. **Nursing Science Quarterly, 5,** 13-18.

Popper, K.R. (1965). **Conjectures and refutations: The growth of scientific knowledge**. New York: Harper Torchbooks.

Rogers, M.E. (1970). **An introduction to the theoretical basis of nursing**. Philadelphia: FA Davis.

Rogers, M.E. (1990). Nursing: Science of unitary, irreducible, human beings: Update 1990. In E.A.M. Barrett (Ed.), **Visions of Rogers' science-based nursing** (pp. 5-11). New York: National League for Nursing.

Roy, C. (1976). **Introduction to nursing: An adaptation model**. Englewood Cliffs, NJ: Prentice-Hall.

Roy, C. (1988). An explication of the philosophical assumptions of the Roy adaptation model. **Nursing Science Quarterly, 1,** 26-34.

Roy, C., & Andrews, H.A. (1991). **The Roy adaptation model: The definitive statement**. Norwalk, CT: Appleton & Lange.

Salsberry, P. (1994). A philosophy of nursing: What is it? What is it not? In J.F. Kikuchi & H. Simmons (Eds.), **Developing a philosophy of nursing** (pp. 11-19). Thousand Oaks, CA: Sage.

Seaver, J.W., & Cartwright, C.A. (1977). A pluralistic foundation for training early childhood professionals. **Curriculum Inquiry, 7,** 305-329.

Watson, J. (1985). **Nursing: Human science and human care: A theory of nursing**. Norwalk, CT: Appleton-Century-Crofts.

Chapter 2
Knowledge Development for Nursing: A Process
Imogene M. King

My analysis of the scientific evolution in formalizing knowledge for nursing has led me to identify a process for developing scientific knowledge. This process is shown in **Figure 1**.

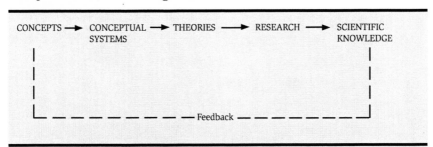

Figure 1: Knowledge development for nursing: A process.

I regard **Figure 1** as a kind of functional connection between concepts that may lead to scientific knowledge and a process for identifying phenomena from the perspective of nursing. This conceptualization provides a map with different roads to travel to arrive at scientific knowledge for nursing. Prior to discussing the components and definitions of terms in **Figure 1**, I would like to discuss some of my philosophical assumptions about human knowing and human beings.

Philosophic Assumptions

Historically, epistemologists and philosophers of science have proposed different assumptions about the nature of knowledge and ways to discover scientific knowledge. Epistemology and philosophy of science, which are two branches of philosophy, are distinct yet related in that each deals with knowledge. For example, epistemology is a philosophic investigation into human knowing and analysis of the various ways of knowing. An exploration of philosophy of science revealed changes about the nature of and methods used to develop scientific knowledge (Suppe, 1989).

My approach to identify essential knowledge for nursing began in the 1960s when my view of science changed while studying systems research. The systems movement in science gained momentum in the 1950s, although its roots date to an earlier period. This movement refuted logical positivism and reductionism and proposed the idea of "perspectivism" in knowledge development. Von Bertalanffy (1968) was credited with originating the idea of a "general system theory." He defined general system theory as a "general science of wholeness: systems of elements in mutual interaction" (p.37).

My philosophic position is rooted in general system theory, which guides the study of organized complexity as whole systems. General system theory guided me to focus on knowledge as an information processing, goal seeking, and decision making system.

Major components in nursing as a discipline are knowledge development, knowledge dissemination, and knowledge utilization. General system theory provides one approach to free nurses from the parts versus whole dilemma. General system theory provides a holistic approach for studying nursing as an open system. A system is a set of elements connected by communication links that exhibits goal-directed behavior.

Human beings are open systems who think, who set goals, and who select means to achieve them. Open systems exhibit an exchange of energy and information and are goal-directed. Resources flow into the system as inputs, activities indicate the use of resources, and outputs are generated. Open systems exhibit equifinality in that different means may be used to attain similar goals. When inputs are converted to outputs, transformation takes place. A system is described as a set of relations among the elements, that is, complex interrelationships of social phenomena in natural environments.

My early ideas were rather traditional and centered on sensory and interpersonal perception. Perception and conception are viewed as ongoing and continuous selection of information available in the internal and external environments. Knowledge development not only involves perception and concept formation but also is an active construction and reconstruction through interchange between an individual and the physical and social environments.

My more recent ideas are centered on transactions. Transactions are viewed as a flow of information from the environment through coding, transformation, and processing of sensory, linguistic, and neurophysiological elements, resulting in decision making that leads to human actions. Internal processing of information is relational because mapping occurs between the knower and the known. Individuals organize and relate information from the external environment with the internal environment. Perception, conception, decision, and action constitute complex interrelations in which external data interact with internal factors to transform inputs and are seen as a process of complex organization and construction of knowledge.

One way of knowing is the transformation of sensory data into concepts that are stored in one's memory. Concepts are associated with intellectual knowledge. Another way of gaining knowledge is through the acts of thinking and reasoning, deductively and inductively. Deduction is a process of reasoning from the abstract (general), such as weather, to the concrete (particular), such as rain. Induction is a process of reasoning in which one proceeds from the concrete, such as table, to the abstract, such as furniture. Human beings, therefore, gain knowledge about their world through a relation between the external and internal environments. Individuals exhibit a sense of wonder about their world and ask questions, seek answers, identify problems, and seek resolution. Human beings have an intellect and by nature, they have the desire to know. (King, 1981)

One assumption about human beings is that individuals are in continuous transaction with their internal and external en-vironments. In addition, assumptions are made that individuals are social, spiritual, sentient, and rational human beings who act in situations by perceiving, controlling, and exhibiting purposeful action-oriented behavior over time. Perceptions of individuals and groups influence interactions. Goals, needs, and values of individuals and groups influence transactions made in a variety of situations (King, 1981, p. 145).

Nursing is perceived by me to be a complex, organized whole system, transacting with a variety of whole systems. The domain of nursing assumes person-environment transactions. The domain focus is helping individuals, families, groups, and communities maintain health. This indicates that nursing is a goal-seeking system.

One's observations of the external environment are represented in language. Many difficulties arise in understanding the use of a word, just as disagreements arise from having a different meaning for the same word. Initially, words represent one's concepts, and discussing the words represents one's personal knowledge. Concepts are essential elements in the process for developing scientific knowledge from a nursing perspective (King, 1988).

Concepts

As can be seen in **Figure 1**, my idea of the process of knowledge development starts with concepts. Concepts are defined as abstract ideas that "give meaning to one's perceptions, permit generalizations, and tend to be stored in one's memory for recall and use in new and different situations" (King, 1971, p. 12). A concept is perceived to be the basic unit of the mind just as the cell is the basic unit of the body (King, 1975, p. 33). Concepts are abstract representations of an individual's comprehension of persons, objects, and events.

Comprehension of a concept is called connotation or intention, that is, we know the essential characteristics (attributes) that tell us the nature or essence of the concept. An extension of a concept is called denotation. Denotation is not the concept but rather the objects to which the concept refers. For example, the characteristics of chair, which are material, nonliving, nonsentient, and substance, represent one's comprehension. Extension means all of the objects to which the idea of chair refers, such as patio chair or upholstered chair (King, 1975).

Concepts categorize one's knowledge and also describe and explain knowledge relevant for a discipline. Concepts represent essential elements that an object, a person, or an event have in common with other persons, objects, and events. Concepts are classified as abstract, such as health, environment, person, and as concrete, such as hair, trees, bones. Concepts are open-ended in a continuous process of expanding one's knowledge.

Several functions of concepts have been suggested. For example, concepts mark off events into categories that tell us more about a subject. Concepts help one analyze events to search for relationships. Concepts are tested and modified in one's experience. They serve as a guide for systematic observation of the concrete world. When tested in research, concepts result in scientific knowledge (King, 1975).

Several nurses have published information about concepts and agree that they are the building blocks for theory construction and testing (Chinn & Jacobs, 1987; King, 1971, 1975, 1988; Norris, 1982; Parse, 1981; Walker & Avant, 1988; Watson, 1985). Concepts, definitions, and propositions that link the concepts have been discussed consistently as major elements in theory construction. Concepts represent substantive knowledge, whereas process represents relationships about ways to use knowledge. Concepts help us identify nursing's phenomena.

Concepts structure the domain of knowledge in a discipline. The structure is identified in the published conceptual systems of the discipline.

Conceptual Systems

The terms conceptual framework, conceptual model, theoretical framework, and conceptual system have been used interchangeably in nursing's literature. My preference as we move into the twenty-first century is to use the term "conceptual system" because the word "system" is a symbol commonly used in all aspects of human activities, in science, and in nursing. For example, a systems framework for change within a neonatal intensive care unit (NICU) was proposed by nurses, who implemented a plan to assist parents interact with their newborns within the hospital system (Norris & Hoyer, 1993). Furthermore, systems approach was used to implement case management in a community health environment (Hampton, 1994; Sowell & Lowenstein, 1994).

A conceptual system is a set of concepts that are defined and linked by broad generalizations constructed by an individual for a purpose. Generally, the functions of a conceptual system are: (a) to provide a way to organize a multitude of facts into meaningful wholes; (b) to provide a common theoretical basis for communications and relationships in a field of study; (c) to direct attention to processes and relationships which are a guarantee for continued learning; (d) to guide one to look for specific facts and their relationships; and (e) to order knowledge for use in a variety of settings (King, 1995).

A conceptual system identifies relevant concepts that describe the structure and focus of a discipline. My analysis of published conceptual systems yielded some of the concepts deemed essential knowledge for nursing. Several examples are: Peplau's (1952) interpersonal relations, Roy's (Roy & Roberts, 1981) adaptation, Levine's (1969) conservation principles, King's (1981) transactions, Watson's (1985) caring, and Parse's (1995) human becoming. A conceptual system provides a schema or world view that helps one focus thinking about relevant phenomena and provides direction for the development of specific theories. Theories are not only derived from conceptual systems but can actually suggest concepts or modification of concepts which in turn affect conceptual systems (Frey & Sieloff, 1995).

Theories

The primary function of theory is to describe, explain, and predict phenomena in a discipline. Theory provides a starting point to collect facts in an organized and systematic way. Theory suggests hypotheses to test and research questions to answer. Theory provides one approach to confirm facts in a discipline. The broader the range of specific events it explains, the more powerful the theory. Theory cannot be limited by time and place; the ultimate criterion of a scientific theory is its direction in adding to an understanding of the world in which we live and the complexity of nursing situations in which nurses practice.

A theory is a set of interrelated concepts, definitions, and propositions that present a systematic view of essential elements in a field of inquiry by specifying relations among variables (King, 1981, pp. 141-144). This definition contains components that are similar to other nursing publications about theory (Chinn & Jacobs, 1987; Hardy, 1974; Jacox, 1974; Norris, 1982).

Some theories are represented by models. A model in science is someone's conceptualization of phenomena, invented for a specific purpose. Models suggest theories which correlate patterns in observable data. The organizing function of a model is to relate a large quantity of data in a very few concepts. The analytical function of a model prevents use of vague ideas and requires precise analysis of concepts and related data. Models may represent a theory, a set of concepts, or a process that link some of the concepts in a theory. Models are usually mathematical or schematic.

Conceptual clarity deals with the meaning of the concepts of a theory. The test of a theory is the extent to which it provides direction to look for answers to questions that are important to nursing.

Theories and models provide a guide for selection of phenomena to be studied. Phenomena guide the selection of the methods of inquiry and data collection techniques to describe, explain, and predict patterns of relations of phenomena in natural situations. Theory is an abstraction that implies prediction based in research. Theory without research and research without some theoretical basis will not build scientific knowledge for a discipline.

Research

The theory-research movement in nursing indicates multiple ideas and different approaches to describe and explain nursing phenomena. The findings from research help to build, test, and refine theory regardless of the use of induction or deduction, qualitative or quantitative methods.

Research is defined as an organized, systematic, and formal process to solve specific problems or answer specific questions resulting in new knowledge or new relationships among phenomena in a discipline (Kerlinger, 1973; Polit & Hungler, 1983; Waltz, Strickland, & Lenz, 1984).

Historically, nurses have followed the rather traditional restrictive methods of research. The methods and data collection techniques of the 1990s are varied, and some are identified with specific conceptual systems (e.g., Parse, 1987; Watson, 1985). The complexity of nursing as an open system demands more than one methodological approach to nursing research. The problems identified and the questions to be answered guide the selection of the method and data collection techniques necessary to solve the problems or answer the questions. Individual nurses have developed research programs to build knowledge in an area of interest. Some nurses have formed groups with common research interests to advance nursing knowledge. Theory construction and testing in research is one approach to generate scientific knowledge in a field of inquiry. What, then, constitutes proper science for building scientific knowledge for nursing?

Scientific Knowledge

Simply, the word science means to know. All science begins with observations. Some science begins with hunches or with a change in a model. One of the aims of science is to explain natural phenomena. Philosophers have debated the nature of science for centuries. Methods of science have been widely discussed and are associated with one's philosophy.

Scientific knowledge does not come in a neat package. A variety of approaches to develop scientific knowledge may be used. My approach, initially, began with some hunches about nursing based on seeking answers to such questions as: Who are nurses? A simple answer was that they are human beings. Other questions were: What are nurses' functions? and Where do they perform their functions? Subsequent to a review of the literature, I was able to identify some comprehensive concepts that consistently appeared in the literature by means of content analysis. These concepts formed the beginning of my conceptualization of nursing.

Scientific knowledge is often equated with scientific method but they are distinct entities. Methods provide a way to select appropriate techniques to collect data about phenomena of interest to nursing. Scientific knowledge results from use of scientific methods in studying natural phenomena.

Summary

The terms concept, conceptual system, model, theory, research, and scientific knowledge have been defined. In addition, an overview of my philosophic assumptions about knowledge development and about human beings has been presented. Concepts have been described as one approach to identify substantive knowledge deemed relevant for nursing and as the essential elements in a conceptual system. Conceptual systems are designed and used to provide structure to organize knowledge in a discipline. I have suggested that conceptual system is a common term that may be used in nursing's scientific movement to replace conceptual framework, conceptual model, and theoretical framework. Theories are often derived from conceptual systems. Theories offer guidance in answering research questions and in hypothesis-testing. Phenomena to be studied determine the research methods and data collection techniques to be used. Research that tests theories in nursing and that builds theory from research generates scientific knowledge for the discipline.

References

Chinn, P.L., & Jacobs, M.K. (1987). **Theory and nursing: A systematic approach** (2nd ed.). St. Louis, MO: Mosby.

Frey, M.A., & Sieloff, C.L. (Eds.). (1995). **Advancing King's systems framework and theory of nursing.** Thousand Oaks, CA: Sage.

Hampton, C.C. (1994). King's theory of goal attainment as a framework for managed care implementation in a hospital setting. **Nursing Science Quarterly, 7,** 170-173.

Hardy, M.E. (1974). Theories: Components, development, evaluation. **Nursing Research, 23,** 100-107.

Jacox, A. (1974). Theory construction in nursing: An overview. **Nursing Research, 23,** 4-13.

Kerlinger, F.N. (1973). **Foundations of behavioral research** (2nd ed.). New York: Holt, Rinehart & Winston.

King, I.M. (1971). **Toward a theory for nursing: General concepts of human behavior.** New York: John Wiley.

King, I.M. (1975). A process for developing concepts for nursing through research. In P. J. Verhonick (Ed.), **Nursing Research I** (pp. 25-43). Boston: Little Brown.

King, I.M. (1981). **A theory for nursing: Systems, concepts and process.** Albany, NY: Delmar.

King, I.M. (1988). Concepts: Essential elements of theories. **Nursing Science Quarterly, 1,** 22-25.

King, I.M. (1995). A systems framework for nursing. In M.A. Frey & C.L. Sieloff (Eds.), **Advancing King's systems sage framework and theory of nursing** (pp. 14-22). Thousand Oaks, CA.

Levine, M.E. (1969). **Introduction to clinical nursing.** Philadelphia: F.A. Davis.

Norris, C.M. (1982). **Concept clarification in nursing.** Rockville, MD: Aspen.

Norris, D.V., & Hoyer, R.J. (1993). Dynamism in practice: Parenting within King's framework. **Nursing Science Quarterly, 6,** 79-85.

Parse, R.R. (1981). **Man-living-health: A theory of nursing.** Albany, NY: Delmar.

Parse, R.R. (1987). **Nursing science: Major paradigms, theories, and critiques.** Philadelphia: Saunders.

Parse, R.R. (Ed.). (1995). **Illuminations: The human becoming theory in practice and research.** New York: National League for Nursing Press.

Peplau, H.E. (1952). **Interpersonal relation in nursing.** New York: G.P. Putnam's Sons.

Polit, D.F., & Hungler, B.F. (1983). **Nursing research** (2nd ed.). Philadelphia: Lippincott.

Roy, C., & Roberts, S.L. (1981). **Theory construction in nursing: An adaptation model.** Englewood Cliffs, NJ: Prentice-Hall.

Sowell, R.L., & Lowenstein, G. (1994). King's theory as a framework for linking theory to practice. **Nursing Connections, 1(3),** 19-31.

Suppe, F. (1989). **The semantic conception of theories and scientific realism.** Urbana, IL: University of Illinois Press.

Von Bertalanffy, L. (1968). **General system theory: Foundations, development, applications.** New York: George Braziller.

Walker, L.C., & Avant, K.C. (1988). **Strategies for theory construction in nursing** (2nd ed.). Norwalk, CT: Appleton & Lange.

Waltz, C.F., Strickland, O.L., & Lenz, E.R. (1984). **Measurement in nursing research.** Philadelphia: F. A. Davis.

Watson, J. (1985). **Nursing: Human science and human caring.** Norwalk, CT: Appleton-Century-Crofts.

Chapter 3
Terminology in Structuring and Developing Nursing Knowledge
Hesook Suzie Kim

Philosophic Orientation

My approach to the development of nursing knowledge is based on the belief that knowledge development in a discipline requires a metaparadigmatic structure specific to that discipline. Such a structure functions as an analytical framework for (a) orienting the discipline's cognitive interests, (b) selecting and determining the locus of interest for knowledge generation, and (c) critique of the nature and content of knowledge development within a discipline. It is also important to note that nursing knowledge refers to the knowledge in the public sphere, not what exists within the minds of specific individual nurses or is used in specific instances of nursing practice. Although I believe that one of the modes through which nursing knowledge is generated is by tapping such individualistic, incidental, and highly private knowledge, any discourse on nursing epistemology must be confined to the disciplinary knowledge in the public sphere. As such, the terminology offered in this chapter centers around a specific metaparadigmatic structure proposed for nursing knowledge with an orientation to systematizing the disciplinary knowledge.

Nursing's knowledge development during the past two decades has followed multiple paths shaded by differing commitments to various philosophies of science, especially to two opposing philosophies of positivism and antipositivism, especially epistemological relativism. On one hand is a continuing effort exerted by many nursing scientists to produce and accumulate theories and empirical work in the tradition of *hard/natural* sciences, and on the other is a movement to develop nursing knowledge with an orientation inherent in the *soft or interpretive* human sciences legacy. As suggested by Stevenson and Woods (1986), nursing has embraced such pluralism without a view toward reconciliation. As this scene of pluralism within nursing's scientific community has produced separate camps and rival knowledge claims, there certainly is a need to develop an integrative and synthesizing framework for nursing epistemology. My premise for this chapter thus rests with this need and adopts the spirit of what Alexander and Colomy (1992) called a postpositivistic approach. In line with this approach, critical realism and metatheory are believed to articulate the epistemological orientations undergirding the terminology offered in this chapter.

A postpositivistic approach is an alternative philosophic model of epistemology that views knowledge development and progress in terms of "elaboration, proliferation, revision, reconstruction, tradition-creation, and tradition-deconstruction" (Alexander & Colomy, 1992, p. 38), and can be envisioned to encompass both critical realism and metatheoretical posture. This approach, therefore, requires a commitment to an ontological and epistemological orientation that allows reconciliations among alternative scientific approaches as well as to an over-arching concern for a disciplinary-wide knowledge development. In nursing at present we need to adopt this postpositivistic approach with commitment to critical realism and metatheory as the perspective for assessing, reassessing, and reconstructing our knowledge development.

Critical Realism

The ontological and epistemological grounding I propose addresses the specific nature of nursing epistemology as a human practice discipline. Inasmuch as nursing knowledge is concerned with human phenomena regardless of whether one considers those phenomena as atomistic or holistic and also is concerned with human practice that requires intersubjective ("human-to-human") connections in a service framework, the objects of epistemological attention in nursing need to be considered from the perspective of human "knowing" both in the context of human agency embedded in the phenomena of interest and of human inquiry oriented to knowledge generation. This means that the philosophic position must be able to accommodate this complexity at a metatheoretical level.

My perspective of critical realism is a reconciliation of two philosophies: (a) epistemological realism, which asserts that the nature of the being and the objects of knowledge exist and act (that is, "endure and operate") independently of the human's inquiring activity in terms of both sense-experiences and thoughts (Bhaskar, 1986; Layder, 1990), and (b) emancipatory epistemology, which accepts on one hand, the fragility and persistence of human subjectivity that produces individualistic, selective, and sometimes unique perceptions, cognition, and interpretations; and on the other hand, the possibility and feasibility of intersubjective understandings and agreements that are founded on what Bhaskar (1986) calls "emancipatory reason" applied to human sciences. It provides a foundation upon which nursing as a discipline will seek "truth claims" relevant to nursing's epistemic needs and engage in continuous critique of truth claims for validation. Bhaskar (1986) explains a truth claim as follows:

> A truth claim typically involves both prescriptive or imperative ("act on X") and a descriptive or evidential ("X is grounded, warranted, justified") component or dimension. What distinguishes truth claims in science from those in ordinary life is not their logical structure, but the nature of their evidential requirements, which incorporate various logical, empirical, inter- and intra-theoretical controls; the object or referent of the truth claim, which is characteristically a causal structure or explanatory mechanism; the persons (and communities) to which the claim is made and presented for redemption and ratification; and the sorts of uses to which the claim, if it is both validated and true, can be put. (p. 183)

Therefore, critical realism leads to a view of nursing knowledge that needs to be evolutionary and critical in that the discipline's truth claims at a given space-time should be considered revisional and tentative, and must be continuously subjected to critical and emancipatory evaluations for self-reflective corrections both at the disciplinary and individual scientist levels. Since critical realism as an epistemological philosophy for a human practice science is utopian to a degree, the knowledge-work (i.e., scientific practice and inquiry) in the discipline has to focus not only on producing specific knowledge important for the discipline but also on criticizing and evaluating such products. Hence, there is a congruence between upholding this philosophy and having the metatheoretical orientation regarding nursing knowledge development.

Metatheoretical Orientation

My concerns and expositions regarding knowledge development in nursing have focused on what Toulmin (1972) called the deep structure of a discipline, hence the metatheory. The deep structure of a discipline refers not only to the conceptual map of the discipline but also to how that map is revised, expanded, and refined. A metatheoretical orientation in nursing knowledge development thus has to do with theoretical meta-analysis, focusing on a systematic study of the nature of knowledge, knowledge cumulation, and epistemological movements of the discipline (Ritzer, 1992). The aim in focusing on nursing metatheory as a part of my intellectual and theoretical pursuits has been to address the need to systematize and scrutinize products of nursing's scientific attention. This effort in metatheory is oriented to assessing the degree of maturity, comprehensiveness, and completeness in nursing's knowledge development and the modes with which it is progressing.

Thus, terminology in nursing knowledge development required with this orientation encompasses a language system necessary to understand the deep structure of nursing epistemology, transcending and going beyond any language system specific to distinct paradigms and theories. As metatheory presupposes the possibility of theoretical pluralism, the terminology in the metatheory of nursing must allow for such multiplicity. In addition, in order for any metatheoretical work to produce coherent analysis, the metatheoretical orientation must also coincide with an ontological/epistemological posture that allows for reflexivity and critique, hence my orientation in *critical realism*. Metatheoretical orientation is thus concerned with what Schwab (1963) called the problems of the substantive structures of a discipline: (a) the problem inherent in identification of the conceptual structure of a discipline; (b) the problem of ephemeral character of knowledge developed within a given substantive structure; and (c) the problem of the "syntactical" structure of a discipline. These problems articulated by Schwab in the 1960s take on a much more complex turn for consideration when we pose them for the discipline of nursing with the posture of critical realism.

Terminology presented in the following sections is organized into two sets: basic terminology and terminology in a metaparadigm. The *basic terminology* refers to a set of terms that are generic in the discourse of nursing epistemology, while the *terminology in a metaparadigm* presents terms that are specific to my metaparadigmatic structure for nursing knowledge. The presentation of the definitions are drawn from my previous publications (Kim, 1983, 1987, 1989, 1993a, 1993b and 1994) and elaborated further in this chapter.

Basic Terminology

I consider the basic terms generic in the discourse of nursing epistemology as those referring to accepted ideas (i.e., those I understand to have attained a level of consensus even among different scientific camps in nursing) about analytical constructs commonly used in talking about nursing knowledge and its development.

Phenomenon and Nursing Phenomenon

The term phenomenon designates an aspect of reality existing as a pre-linguistic entity and adopting a linguistic meaning upon human perception, recognition, and experience. All aspects of reality in this sense represent either separate, multiple phenomena or a single phenomenon. Hence, as a pre-linguistic entity, a phenomenon such as a girl's smile or a patient's suffering presents itself and exists regardless of whether we have a name for it or realize its existence. Although a girl's smile is readily perceptible and recognizable even though it is open to different interpretations, a patient's suffering requires secondary means to recognize its existence. Furthermore, in general epistemology and science, as well as in ordinary life, we have developed and continue to develop ways to demarcate reality into separate entities through both formal and informal descriptive and classificatory schemes. A given phenomenon can have multiple meanings according to the context within which the phenomenon is perceived and interpreted. Multiple meanings of a phenomenon do not change the essence of the phenomenon: the essence is given different meanings according to different "descriptive" schemata used for interpretation and classification of the essence.

Nursing phenomenon then refers to a phenomenon that pertains to nursing's epistemic interest. Of all phenomena possible in reality, nursing as a discipline considers certain phenomena to require understanding and explanation in order to improve the nature of nursing practice, that is, from the nursing perspective. Thus, the designation of phenomena as nursing depends on the nature of nursing practice mandated and/or institutionalized within a given society. Since social mandates regarding the nature of disciplines, and practice disciplines are especially fluid and changeable, nursing phenomena designated as such at any given time and place require a certain level of intersubjective consensus within the discipline. Nursing phenomena are viewed to exist in general in the realms of clients, client-nurse encounters, nursing practitioners, and nursing-practice environment.

Concept

The term concept refers to a linguistic label given to things, events, ideas, and other realities we perceive and think about. "A concept is a symbolic statement describing a phenomenon or a class of phenomena. Therefore, it is expressed by a definition" (Kim, 1983, p. 8). A concept is derived through either individual or collective cognitive processing to name aspects of reality and refers to either a single, unique entity or a class of phenomena having the same properties that are specified in the definition. In sciences, concepts referring to classes of phenomena rather than a single, unique entity are used to communicate about phenomena of concern in theoretical statements or in empirical work. Nursing concepts are those pertaining to nursing phenomena and are developed through the process of conceptualization within the discipline of nursing. Hence, concepts and their definitions require intersubjective understanding and recognition to be applied in scientific work.

There are many different ways of categorizing concepts according to their characteristics, for example into process versus property concepts. Since nursing is basically concerned with two kinds of reality—(a) the state of things and (b) the way things happen—nursing concepts may be classified as *process* and *property* types for analytic purposes (Kim, 1983). Concepts also can be concrete concepts pertaining to specific, particular phenomena or abstract concepts referring to classes of phenomena not tied to specific time and space. However, scientific concepts are generally abstract because the basic aim of science is to gain knowledge about classes of phenomena.

Theory

The term theory is defined as a set of theoretical statements that provides an understanding and explanation about a class or classes of phenomena. Theory provides a systematic basis for sorting out regularities from irregularities and a heuristic basis of explanation regarding selected aspects of reality. Theoretical statements in a theory are specifications of relationships among conceptual elements of a theory, and can be either descriptive or explanatory. A theory is, therefore, characterized by its logical form, which ties together its theoretical statements; its scope of applicability; and its heuristic form in terms of understanding, explanation, causality, and prescription.

Theoretical framework is a term used to denote a general perspective of a logically coherent integration of theoretical positions regarding a set of concepts, which becomes the basis for developing a system of related theories. Theoretical frameworks specify the nature of theoretical relationships among concepts at a general level and the scope within which such theoretical relationships are applicable.

Conceptual framework refers to a general perspective of organizing and classifying concepts into a relevance structure. Hence, conceptual frameworks contain definitions of concepts and rationales for bringing selected concepts together into relevant structures. Thus, they are pre-theoretical but systematic and analytically coherent, and they contain descriptive statements.

Paradigm

The term paradigm, made fashionable by Kuhn (1970), is used in a restricted sense to refer to a specific scientific tradition in terms of: (a) major form(s) of explanation/heuristic espoused, (b) the perspective with which essential phenomena of concern to a discipline are conceptualized, and (c) the specific commitment to scientific method(s) for knowledge development. In nursing, knowledge is being developed from various paradigmatic orientations, for example, systems, biobehavioral, holistic, and phenomenological paradigms.

Metaparadigm

The term metaparadigm refers to an analytical framework for a discipline that specifies the guidelines, principles, and procedures with which the phenomena of concern for the discipline are delineated and articulated. The metaparadigm transcends any and all specific theoretical or paradigmatic orientations that may exist within a discipline's scientific culture, and provides a way of organizing conceptual clusters of a discipline (Kim, 1989). It represents analytical and organizational schemata for a discipline's knowledge. Metaparadigm is "an organizing framework that permits scientists to impose order on the phenomena of interest" and is "a necessary prerequisite for developing theories and theoretical models" (Kim, 1987, p. 100). It is a framework at a disciplinary level by which relevant phenomena and associated concepts are selected and differentiated within the perspective of a discipline. The metaparadigm for nursing provides the basis from which nursing scientists select and study phenomena of concern, and systematize knowledge within the discipline of nursing.

Terminology in a Metaparadigm for Nursing

Terminology presented in this section is composed of the terms specific to a metaparadigm for nursing developed in my earlier work, which has been referred to as *a typology of four domains of nursing*. This typology of four domains of nursing has been proposed as a conceptual map of nursing concepts and as a sensitizing, analytical scheme for nursing research. The typology is also a framework for structuring nursing knowledge by which the status of nursing knowledge development may be assessed and evaluated.

Domain

Shapere (1977) defines a scientific domain as being composed of related items for scientific investigation, constituting a unified subject matter that poses important problem(s) for scientific investigation and having the quality of readiness in a scientific sense to deal with the problem the subject matter presents. Following this suggested use of the term domain referring to a "field" of related items representing a unified subject matter, nursing concepts are differentiated into four separate domains. Although the term domain is commonly used to refer to knowledge in different disciplines, such as nursing domain, medical domain, and sociological domain, in this typology domains are used to refer more strictly to the locus of nursing phenomena with the assumption that nursing phenomena pertaining to a specific locus (such as client, nurse, nurse-client, or environment) represent specific unified subject matter.

The domains in the typology point to "four spheres of the empirical world in which nursing-relevant phenomena could be located" (Kim, 1987, p. 101), and at the same time orient scientists to the specific nature of the subject matter in the domains. In this sense, the nursing domain as a disciplinary domain is composed of four sub-domains specified in the typology as the client domain, the client-nurse domain, the practice domain, and the environment domain. "Although [this] differentiation of the nursing 'domain' into four separate domains is appropriate, the separate domains may still need to be combined into a larger domain if the larger domain, specifying the discipline, poses a distinct epistemological problem that cannot be independently addressed by the subdomain solutions" (Kim, 1987, p. 100).

The Client Domain

This domain is defined as the area of epistemological focus on phenomena in the client. Hence, the focus is on *the client*. The emphasis is on gaining knowledge about human phenomena (that is, phenomena of the client) from the nursing perspective. Nursing phenomena and concepts in the client domain are considered to belong to four classes: (a) essentialistic phenomena/concepts, (b) developmental phenomena/concepts, (c) problematic phenomena/concepts, and (d) health-care experiential phenomena/concepts.

Essentialistic phenomena/concepts are those pertaining to essential human characteristics, processes, and experiences important and critical for nursing to have knowledge about in developing the knowledge of nursing clients. *Developmental phenomena/concepts* refer specifically to those human characteristics, processes, and experiences in the context of human development and growth. Inasmuch as knowledge about various aspects of life-span development is critical for nursing, developmental phenomena/concepts, although essentialistic in nature, are separately conceptualized to highlight this need. *Problematic phenomena/concepts* refer to those states, events, processes, and experiences in humans that require specific nursing attention for care and therapy. Hence, the term problematic is used to mean problematic to nursing, requiring nursing solutions. *Health-care experiential phenomena/concepts* consist of particular human states, events, processes, and experiences that are confined to clients in health-care contexts. Thus, this class of phenomena/concepts is generic and existentially possible only in being clients of health-care.

The Client-Nurse Domain

The client-nurse domain is designated as the area of study in nursing addressing phenomena arising out of encounters between client and nurse. Hence, the focus is on *the client-nurse in engagement.* The client-nurse domain consists of phenomena/concepts pertaining to contacts, communication, and interaction between client and nurse that occur in the process of providing nursing care. Phenomena in the client-nurse domain belong spatially and temporally to both participants in a joined context, that is, belong to both the client and nurse collectively. Thus, such phenomena are distinctively considered in this domain distinguished from phenomena pertaining to clients or nurses separately. Knowledge in the client-nurse domain is essential as nursing uses client-nurse encounters as the medium through which nursing care and therapy are delivered to clients.

The Practice Domain

The practice domain is concerned with knowledge about phenomena particular to the nurse who is engaged in nursing practice. Hence, the focus is on *the nurse.* Nursing practice is viewed with the focus on the nurse as an agent of action involved in both the phases of deliberation and enactment (Kim, 1994). Nursing practice also involves cognitive, behavioral, and social aspects of professional actions assumed by a nurse in addressing clients and clients' nursing problems. Knowledge in the practice domain is essential for nursing as the knowledge about clients and client-nurse has to be put into use by nurses in actual instances of practice. Knowledge about processes and experiences of practice can be developed by focusing on phenomena in the practice domain. This domain is specifically important for human practice disciplines such as nursing. Nursing's particular practice problems, issues, and experiences belong as subject matter within this domain. Knowledge in this domain is especially critical since nursing practice can also be conceptualized to pertain to three dimensions: scientific, ethical, and aesthetic (Kim, 1993b).

The Environment Domain

The environment domain is designated as an area of study in nursing that focuses on contextual aspects of human living and nursing care. Hence, the focus is *the environment.* "Environment is defined as the entity that exists external to a person or to humanity, conceived either as a whole or as that containing many distinct elements" (Kim, 1983, p. 80). Therefore, in this definition, the elements often delineated as internal environment or internal milieu in the literature are excluded from the concept of environment. Environmental phenomena/concepts may be described in terms of spatial, temporal, and qualitative characteristics and with respect to physical, social, and symbolic dimensions. For nursing, phenomena/concepts in the environment domain are of interest so long as they provide understandings, insights, illustrations, and explanations regarding phenomena in the client, client-nurse, and practice domains. One specific area of importance for knowledge development relevant to nursing pertains to phenomena in the health-care environment. Since clients' experiences, client-nurse encounters, and nursing practice take place in the health-care environment, it is important to gain specific knowledge regarding the health-care environment.

Conclusion

Two sets of terminology described in this chapter provide clarification of terms necessary in metatheoretical analysis of nursing knowledge. Metatheoretical analysis of nursing knowledge involves examinations and analyses of the progress nursing as a discipline is making in systematizing and developing its knowledge-base. There are three distinct activities involved in metatheoretical work in nursing epistemology:

- Increasing specification and consolidation of concepts for their relevance and importance for knowledge development in the nursing context with a view toward a comprehensive mapping of the metaparadigm of nursing knowledge
- Meta-analysis of the nature of theoretical thinking in nursing with an emphasis on identifying coherence and linkages among philosophies of ontology, epistemology, and nursing, metaparadigm focus, paradigm orientation, and theoretical contents (Kim, 1989, 1993a)
- Examination of philosophic, scientific, and social forces and movements, both internal and external to the discipline of nursing, that influence the development of nursing knowledge and nursing practice

These are necessary activities for developing nursing's epistemological sensibility and gaining understanding about the discipline's progress in systematizing its knowledge base. Terminology presented in this chapter is a useful starting point for metatheoretical analysis in charting nursing epistemology's developmental course.

References

Alexander, J.C., & Colomy, P. (1992). Traditions and competition: Preface to a postpositivist approach to knowledge cumulation. In G. Ritzer (Ed.), **Metatheorizing** (pp. 27-52). Newbury Park, CA: Sage.

Bhaskar, R. (1986). **Scientific realism and human emancipation**. London: Verso.

Kim, H.S. (1983). **The nature of theoretical thinking in nursing**. Norwalk, CT: Appleton-Century-Crofts.

Kim, H.S. (1987). Structuring the nursing knowledge system: A typology of four domains. **Scholarly Inquiry for Nursing Practice: An International Journal, 1**, 99-110.

Kim, H.S. (1989). Theoretical thinking in nursing: Problems and prospects. In J. Akinsanya (Ed.), **Recent advances in nursing: Models of nursing** (pp. 106-122). Edinburgh, Scotland: Churchill Livingstone.

Kim, H.S. (1993a). Identifying alternative linkages among philosophy, theory and method in nursing science. **Journal of Advanced Nursing, 18**, 793-800.

Kim, H.S. (1993b). Response to "Nursing as aesthetic experience and the notion of practice." **Scholarly Inquiry for Nursing Practice: An International Journal, 7**, 279-282.

Kim, H.S. (1994). Practice theories in nursing and a science of nursing practice. **Scholarly Inquiry for Nursing Practice: An International Journal, 8**, 145-158.

Kuhn, T. (1970). **Structure of scientific revolutions**. Chicago: University of Chicago Press.

Layder, D. (1990). **The realist image in social science**. London: Macmillan.

Ritzer, G. (1992). Metatheorizing in sociology: Explaining the coming of age. In G. Ritzer (Ed.), **Metatheorizing** (pp. 7-26). Newbury Park, CA: Sage.

Schwab, J.J. (1963). Structure of the disciplines: Meanings and significances. In G.W. Ford & L. Pugno (Eds.), **The structure of knowledge and the curriculum** (pp. 6-49). Chicago: Rand McNally & Company.

Shapere, D. (1977). Scientific theories and their domains. In F. Suppe (Ed.), **The structure of scientific theories** (2nd ed., pp. 518-599). Urbana, IL: University of Chicago Press.

Stevenson, J.S., & Woods, N.F. (1986). Nursing science and contemporary science: Emerging paradigms. In G.E. Sorensen (Ed.), **Setting the agenda for the year 2000: Knowledge development in nursing** (pp. 6-20). Kansas City, MO: American Academy of Nursing.

Toulmin, S. (1972). **Human understanding. Vol. 1, The collective use and evolution of concepts**. Princeton, NJ: Princeton University Press.

Chapter 4
Nursing Theory and Metatheory
Joyce J. Fitzpatrick

Definitions of Terms and Rationale

A theory is a set of interrelated concepts, based on assumptions, woven together through a set of propositional statements. Theories are used to symbolically describe reality; they reflect an interpretation of reality. This view of theory is consistent with the Oxford English Dictionary (1970) definition of theory as "a scheme or system of ideas or statements held as an explanation or account of a group of facts or phenomena." Further, this definition of theory is consistent with the philosophic basis of symbolic logic, first proposed by Whitehead and Russell in 1910 (Brown, 1977). Kuhn's description of the development of scientific revolutions through a process of theory testing in normal science is an important foundation for the views included here. According to Kuhn (1962), as the basic assumptions or conceptual boundaries change, new ways to interpret observations emerge.

Dimensions of Theories

Theories can be described and defined along various dimensions. One of these dimensions is the level of abstraction embedded in the concepts and theoretical statements inherent in the theory. Another is the degree of generalizability of the theory. Using both of these criteria together leads to development of a relationship between the various levels of theory in nursing. Thus, a continuum of theory could be developed with broad grand or metatheories at one level, and very specific focused theories at the other extreme.

"Meta," a prefix from the Greek, has been used in sciences to form a designation for a higher science (actual or hypothetical) of the same nature but dealing with ulterior and/or more fundamental problems (Oxford English Dictionary, 1970), Thus, using this criterion as the distinguishing dimension, metatheory can be defined as a higher level of theory.

One can think of the term "theory" as a general term, including the subset of metatheory, or reserve the label "theory" for a level of conceptualization that is more specific than metatheory. Using this distinction in categorizing nursing conceptualizations, one could conclude that the conceptual models of nursing are generally at the metatheory level. Some of them also include more specific theoretical statements, ones that could best be described as middle-range theory, consisting of a set of relational statements from which testable hypotheses can be derived. One of the issues in the debate and discussions of nursing theories has been related to the inclusion or exclusion of the conceptual models as theory. Of course, consistent conclusions can only be reached if there are consistent definitions of the term theory.

Analysis of Nursing Conceptual Models

In a comprehensive analysis of the majority of the nursing conceptual models, I have argued that these models do, in fact, constitute a level of nursing theory (Fitzpatrick & Whall, 1989). There is, however, a wide range of specificity in the nursing models, with concomitant limits on generalizability. Various examples of nursing metatheory can be identified in the nursing conceptual models, from Nightingale's (1859) focus on the laws of health, to Rogers' (1990) focus on unitary persons, to Newman's (1994) focus on health as expanding consciousness.

My own model is directly derived from Rogers' (1970, 1980, 1983) conceptualization of unitary persons. I regard this "rhythm model" as a level of theory that is less abstract than Rogers' conceptualization. Two approaches were used in deriving the rhythm model. First, research results from a number of studies were examined from the theoretical perspective of Rogers. Although the specific studies were not derived from Rogers' conceptualization, the findings were deemed consistent with Rogers' model. Following this conceptual and theoretical analysis, a number of empirical studies were undertaken to test the propositions derived from Rogers and consistent with the Fitzpatrick rhythm model. Results from these studies were used to further refine the conceptualization. Thus, a combination of deductive and inductive processes was used to further develop the model (Fitzpatrick, 1989).

Using Theory

The belief that theory exists to categorize and explain our world is inherent in my work. Theory alone is not useful. Rather, theory is the use to which the theory is subjected that is significant. Theory exists in nursing to help professionals provide better nursing care, and the test of nursing science, both theory and research, is a test of its applicability to professional practice.

Summary

Definitions of both theory and metatheory have been presented from my particular perspective. General criteria to distinguish levels of theory have been discussed. In addition, the derivation of my own theory, based on Rogers' conceptualization, was outlined.

References

Brown, H. (1977). **Perception, theory and commitment: The new philosophy of science**. Chicago: University of Chicago Press.

Fitzpatrick, J.J. (1989). A life perspective rhythm model. In J.J. Fitzpatrick & A.L. Whall (Eds.), **Conceptual models of nursing: Analysis and application** (2nd ed., pp. 401-407). Norwalk, CT: Appleton and Lange.

Fitzpatrick, J.J., & Whall, A.L. (Eds.). (1989). **Conceptual models of nursing: Analysis and application** (2nd ed.). Norwalk, CT: Appleton and Lange.

Kuhn, T.S. (1962). **The structure of scientific revolutions.** Chicago: University of Chicago Press.

Newman, M.A. (1994). **Health as expanding consciousness** (2nd ed.). New York: National League for Nursing Press.

Nightingale, F. (1859). **Notes on nursing: What it is, and what it is not**. London: Harrison and Sons. [Commemorative edition printed by J. B. Lippincott Company, Philadelphia, 1992.]

Oxford English Dictionary. (1970). Cambridge: Oxford University Press.

Rogers, M.E. (1970). **An introduction to the theoretical basis of nursing**. Philadelphia: F. A. Davis.

Rogers, M.E. (1980). Nursing: A science of unitary man. In J.P. Riehl & C. Roy (Eds.), **Conceptual models for nursing practice** (2nd ed., 329-337). New York: Appleton-Century-Crofts.

Rogers, M.E. (1983). **Science of unitary human beings: A paradigm for nursing**. Unpublished manuscript, New York University, New York, NY.

Rogers, M.E. (1990). Nursing: Science of unitary, irreducible, human beings: Update 1990. In E.A.M. Barrett (Ed.), **Visions of Rogers' science-based nursing** (5-11). New York: National League for Nursing.

Chapter 5
Theoretical Nursing: Definitions and Interpretations

Afaf Ibrahim Meleis

The definitions of key concepts proposed in this chapter reflect the philosophic views that I have adopted, the experiences that I have had, my educational background and the intellectual growth I have experienced over the decades of considering and thinking theory. They are dynamic definitions that will continue to emerge, evolve and be transformed by more study, more experiences, and more reflection on meanings and interpretations.

Philosophic Orientation

Perhaps the most profound influence on the nature of these definitions is my feminist perspective which shapes the very fabric of my tentative realities. My feminist perspective includes recognizing the role of patriarchy in societies in defining knowledge, evaluating knowledge, prioritizing knowledge, and accepting knowledge. It also includes questioning the conditions upon which terms are defined and concepts are refined, and the roles of gendered symbols and metaphors in driving the type of theory and the nature of science that nurses engage in creating. Concepts of objectivity, truth, distancing, and dualism, when considered from a feminist perspective, tend to isolate knowledge from dominant social values, perceived meanings, and agents of knowledge development. I have accepted the view that knowledge has historical and sociopolitical contexts and cannot be developed, refined or understood without those contexts. A feminist perspective provides a platform to reform definitions, to reformulate theoretical goals, and to relocate them within time and socio-cultural and political contexts. I am influenced by such authors as Bleier (1990) in the definitions I offer in the literature about knowledge development.

Another major influence in my thinking of theory is the tradition of symbolic interactionism. Theories evolve and are shaped through interactions with one's environment at large, significant others, and reference groups, in particular. The self influences others and environments inasmuch as it is influenced by others. To understand a human being's responses, a theorist must then access the meanings, the values, and the interpretations of situations embedded in the social world of the individual. These meanings and values ultimately organize and shape individuals' responses. Thoughts, interpretations and actions of individuals continuously and dynamically create perceived realities (Bhimer, 1969; Mead, 1934; Turner, 1968). In particular, my views of the dynamic, evolving, and integrative nature of knowledge and the proactive involvements of agents of knowledge, which include theorists, scientists, clinicians, and the public as participants in the processes of knowledge, are shaped by this philosophic view. Therefore, knowledge is dynamic, always tentative, always evolving, always changing, and never static or complete. There are multiple realities, and there are multiple and various interpretations of these realities. Reality is not illusive, rather it is rich and complex. Much caution needs to be devoted to what labels we choose to use, what meanings we adopt, and what interpretations we opt for. The labels tend to be influenced by some of these realities and in turn, the labels shape these realities.

In defining the major metatheoretical concepts that we are using or should and could use to frame our discipline and determine its boundaries, I assume that the less jargon used, the more we can expect clinicians to participate in knowledge development. Members of the discipline of nursing may benefit from the processes that other disciplines encounter in facilitating progress in developing knowledge and those that have constrained the development of knowledge.

Finally, I believe that when we are not able to articulate our frameworks for observation, action, or interpretation, it s not because we do not have a framework, but rather is most likely that we are not aware or conscious of these frameworks. The danger in our inability to articulate a framework that is guiding our analysis or interpretation is that we may go into "default mode" and may not be aware of it. The default philosophic and theoretic modes are most probably the one that has dominated health care—the biomedical model—or the one that tends to dominate the health system—the economic model. The following definitions reflect my philosophic views within the context of my history and experiences.

Terminology

The Discipline

The discipline of nursing is defined by its domain, its unique perspective, the shared definitions of nursing, and the central roles of its members. A discipline provides a unique way of considering the phenomena that are of interest to its members. Disciplines claim a particular knowledge base as well as ways by which knowledge is obtained and developed. Disciplines are organized to form a structure within academic institutions (Becher & Kogan, 1980). All disciplines are formed around a focal domain, and they have knowledge communities (Oldnall, 1995).

The discipline of nursing includes the content and processes related to the roles that nurses play, such as teacher, administrator, clinician, consultant, researcher, and theoretician. These constitute knowledge communities with a sense of collectivizing. The discipline also includes the theories developed to describe, explain, prescribe, or predict the nature of the phenomena with which members of the discipline deal. In addition, the discipline includes schools of research traditions organized to answer the discipline's problems (Meleis, 1991).

Domains of Knowledge

A domain of knowledge is the crux of the discipline. A domain is the territory that shapes both its theoretical and practical boundaries. These boundaries represent the current state of the investigative interests of the discipline's community. These investigative interests are dynamic and changing, and reflect waves of questions that are significant to members of the discipline and evolve into traditions of research (Laudan, 1977, 1981). There is a dialectical process between the questions investigated, the nature of support for the investigations, which in turn drives the development of more related questions.

The Domain of Nursing

I am influenced in my definition of the domain of nursing by the writings of Kuhn (1970), Merton (1973), Parsons (1951), and Toulmin (1972). The domain of nursing is defined by the phenomena that members of the discipline deal with and are interested in. It contains the major problem areas of the field, those that drive the research questions, as well as the theories developed and the ones to be developed. A domain also reflects the wisdom and the experiences of those who play different roles within the discipline. A domain encompasses the tools used for the development of knowledge.

A domain informs and is informed by clinical practice and research as well as by other roles that members of the discipline may play. A domain does not simply include the results of research projects, theories, or practice. Rather, it encompasses the frameworks that drive nursing research, that shape its theories, and that drive its practice. It is shaped by the units of analysis used to measure phenomena.

Domains are dynamic and responsive to societal needs, to research findings, and to evolving definitions of phenomenon. The nursing domain contains a focus on environments, interactions, human beings, responses to health and illness, relationships, and health.

Philosophy

A philosophy of a discipline encompasses the values, norms, and beliefs that influence the context of its theories and research and the processes utilized in developing them. To speak of nurses' philosophies is to access their orientation to life, their practice, the moral dilemmas they encounter, and the meanings they ascribe to events. A philosophy includes the values that people hold, the beliefs that shape their interactions, and the standards that guide the options they create, as well as the choices they make (Kaplan, 1964).

Paradigm

The concept of paradigm is closely associated with Kuhn (1970), who introduced the concept to the scientific community in an attempt to revise the views of philosophy of science held at that time. Paradigm is defined as a shared framework and a shared view held by members of a discipline about the discipline. Later, Kuhn (1977, p. 297) proposed to replace the concept of paradigm with "disciplinary matrix." A "disciplinary matrix" includes the shared commitment of the community of scholars, the shared symbolic generalizations, the exemplars that constitute the main discipline's problems, and the answers to the main questions. I suggest that the prevailing view in nursing is the definition of paradigm as a school of thought, such as the needs paradigm; a shared set of attributes that identify a particular methodological approach to research, such as the qualitative and quantitative paradigms; and/or a shared central characteristic of the discipline, such as the holistic versus the reductionistic paradigm. Each one of these meanings is characterized by a group of agents, actors, and members of the discipline who tend to share a constellation of values, norms, beliefs, goals, attributes, methods, and views. Therefore, I define paradigm to reflect a number of properties that reflect a community of a discipline's members and a set of properties that describe some aspect of the discipline. For example, the caring paradigm brings images of a number of theorists in nursing who have made significant contributions to defining nursing as caring, and to developing the methodology that respects the assumptions inherent in caring. It also refers to distinguishing assumptions, statements, and the mission inherent in caring.

Paradigm shifts occur when phenomena and questions are considered and analyzed through new lenses and new methods (Kuhn, 1970). Kuhn (1970, 1977) designated disciplines to the preparadigm stage when there is lack of agreement about particular frameworks for knowledge development, priorities, investigation, and ways by which these priorities are actualized. Kuhn's (1970) paradigms evolve after revolutions that proceed from crises of multiplicities to periods of normal science wherever one paradigm dominates and others are disputed.

I propose that the development of the discipline of nursing may have charted a course that was neither revolutionary or evolutionary. There is evidence that the discipline of nursing grew through a process of integration of rejected and accepted theories; old and more contemporary, collaborative and competitive models; and qualitative and quantitative methods. Integration theory for knowledge development does not lead to a paradigm solution, rather it leads to accommodation, refinement, and collaboration in knowledge development, and ultimately to the achievement of a disciplinary status and a position of scholarship (Meleis, 1991). Therefore, nursing is neither at a preparadigmatic nor a paradigmatic state. It is a scholarly discipline reflecting an integrative approach to knowledge development.

Theory

A theory is a mental image of a coherent view of a phenomenon and/or its relationship to other phenomena. Theories are abstract representations of a reality formulated to answer some significant questions. Theory is an organized, coherent, and systematic articulation of a set of statements related to significant questions in a discipline that is communicated in a meaningful whole. Theories have concepts, descriptive statements, prepositions, and a narrative explanation. Theory is an articulation of nursing phenomena developed to describe a phenomenon and provide a framework to anticipate and explain patterns related to the phenomenon. Nursing theories must be communicated in a coherent whole of what is or what could be in relationship to a phenomenon. They address a specific aspect of nursing as they relate to human responses to health and illness. Theories drive inquiry, and they are reservoirs for findings related to phenomena. Theories may be identified in terms of their disciplines, such as the psychological, sociological, or biological nursing theories. Any of these theories could be used to support the mission and the goals of nursing. However, nursing is distinguished from other disciplines by those theories that are related to nursing's central phenomena, such as self-care, comfort, touching, monitoring, presence, supporting, personal resources, living with symptoms, and symptom management, among others. Use of theories of other disciplines may facilitate nursing's mission and achieve nursing goals, but by themselves do not direct nursing's mission or overall goals.

Theories in nursing are tentative, dynamic, changing, and in process. Theories reflect some aspect of reality and include basic truths upon which tentative truths are logically built and prepared. Theories in human science disciplines are placed in historical contexts and, therefore, could be understood in terms of the sociopolitical forces of the period during which the theory was constructed.

Theories are defined in terms of their level of abstraction and scope of explanation as grand, middle range, and narrow range. They are defined in relationship to research as theory-testing or theory-generating research. They are defined in terms of their discipline association as unique (nursing theories), borrowed (psychological, sociological, or biological theories), or derived (maternal role attainment, role supplementation). Barnum (1994) proposed shared theories to substitute the borrowed theories with the assumption that knowledge is shared. Theories are also defined in terms of the type of knowledge reflected, including descriptive, explanatory, and predictive theories. Moreover, they are defined in terms of their content, that is, need, caring, holistic health, interaction, and outcome. Theories are also defined by their authors name, such as King, Orem, and Johnson. Finally, theories are defined in terms of their goals, such as descriptive, practice, or prescriptive theories.

The nature of questions that drive the development of nursing theories changes and evolves to reflect the level of knowledge development. Early theorists attempted to answer questions related to what nursing is. The current generation of theorists are answering questions related to central phenomena in nursing, attainments and developments, and comforting and caring for patients.

In addition, in a humanistic practice discipline, theories must reflect and emanate from the daily practice of nurses. The ultimate goal is to develop theories that maintain, enforce, nurture, stimulate, control, and augment responses to health and illness. These theories could provide guidelines for practice. Therefore, I propose that future theories in nursing will be situational, that is, theories that are defined in terms of their limited historical, environmental and conditional contexts. Generalizations from these theories are limited to these contexts and the limited number of theoretical statements in these theories. Examples of future theories are comfort for vulnerable population, therapeutic touch among low propensity for touch populations, at risk roles and wellness, and transitions into long term institutions. Finally, theories will be less defined by authors (e.g., Roy, King) and more defined by the phenomena of interest (e.g., wound healing, clinical decision, interaction, and disclosure), and cumulatively will be developed by a number of theorists working independently.

Theoretical Thinking

In a human science and a practice discipline, theory development as a goal is secondary to the development of theoretical thinking among members of the knowledge community. The components of theoretical thinking include the processes of analysis of situations, events, and actions that include reflection, connection with other ideas, interpretation, generating meaning, abstracting, comparing, contrasting, and/or utilizing theories to explain situations or guide actions. The strategies of theoretical thinking are to reduce, synthesize, and/or analyze the components. The goals are integrate into more coherent wholes, develop a more coherent view, and create some order related to ideas where none may have existed and/or where pre-existing wholes are not as illuminating as new proposed integrated wholes (Meleis, 1987).

Theoretical thinking should be an integral part of education in the discipline of nursing. It differentiates scholarly practice from practice, scholarly research from research, scholarly utilization of theory from application of theory. It also differentiates stagnant disciplines from those that are dynamic and responsive to society's needs.

Assumptions

Assumptions are those statements that are taken for granted and accepted, the premises upon which concepts are developed, theories evolve, and research is conducted. Assumptions are those statements authors consider to have support for high probability of truth. They are statements that reflect values, beliefs and/or goals related to a concept, theory, discipline, or nursing action. These statements represent the thread that holds different aspects of knowledge together. They represent an author's, clinician's, researcher's, or theorist's biases. Assumptions may be implicit or explicit, that is, they may be clearly stated or they may be inferred from the author's writings. Although assumptions are not advanced for debate or for further analysis or testing, they could be subjected to debate, analysis, or testing by others who question their relevance, authenticity, truth or bias. Assumptions could also be subjected to evaluation, testing, and analyses, using philosophic or theoretic approaches.To understand and interpret a theory or a research finding, assumptions must be carefully uncovered and analyzed. Moreover, the assumptions of the creators of knowledge and those of the consumers of knowledge should be uncovered.

Conceptual Frameworks and Models

A conceptual framework or model is a structure or model that evolves from a theory or a number of theories, built for the purpose of generating questions. It is a mental or physical image of a structure that evolves from a theory or from the integration of a number of theories in some unique way to generate new questions or to view new relationships. The structure revolves around some central nursing phenomena. An example is a conceptual model for social support that reflects and evolves from network theory, bonding theory, and social support theory. Another example is a model for networking and health that is developed from integrating networking theory and a theory for health promotion. A third example is a model of maternal role attainment and social support that reflects maternal role attainment and social support theories. Models have the same structural components as the theory or the theories that they model but have only limited complexity of each concept and the relationships between concepts. According to Kaplan (1964), a model resembles an original system in structural form, but not necessarily in content. Nursing theories are considered models because they were modeled after other theories, such as system adaptation and developmental and symbolic interaction theories. Models are also considered less abstract than theories. They have all the variables in the original theory, but they are closer to reality (Kaplan, 1964).

Conceptual models, theories, conceptual frameworks, and theoretical frameworks have been used to represent distinctly different levels of abstractions, different goals, and different levels of specificity. They have also been used interchangeably (Meleis, 1991). My perspective on the debate about the different meanings of each of these labels is consistent with my philosophical orientation, as stated at the beginning of this chapter. To debate the differences is fruitless and unproductive. I relegate the differences to the multidisciplinary preparation of nursing scholars and to semantics. I take the position that all of the terms have been used interchangeably and that using them interchangeably is inconsequential. I also take the position that a more productive use of the intellectual and theoretical capabilities of nurse scholars is to debate the substantive issues in the discipline. When the domain of nursing has been sufficiently developed and advanced through productive debates, research, and theory development, structural debates could be afforded. There are many examples of theories that have been considered models, concepts, or theories. The extent to which such usage has constrained or facilitated the consequences of knowledge progress is debatable.

Phenomena

Phenomena are things, events, or situations that exist in reality and reflect an aspect of reality. Phenomena are an aspect of that reality colored by the perception of the view of that reality. Phenomena remain phenomena as long as we attach no cognitive, intuitive, or inferential interpretations. The same phenomenon will have different meanings when viewed from different perspectives and through different philosophic and conceptual frameworks. The departure of high school graduates from their parents' home to colleges and new living arrangements is a phenomenon in the U.S. It is one that is interpreted as normal, a milestone, expected, and accepted. The same phenomenon in other countries is considered abnormal and is not accepted. When phenomena are recognized as phenomena, when they are related to other classes of phenomena, and when they are shaped and given some form and some order, they become closer to a concept.

Concepts

Concepts are abstract, mental images of phenomena with a label that distinguishes them from other phenomena or classes of phenomena. Concepts reflect sense observations, inferences, intuitive leaps, and a systematic representation of phenomena. Concepts vary in levels of abstraction (transitions, postpartum transitions) and degrees of specificity (symptom management, management of shortness of breath). The labels selected to reflect and depict phenomena become vital in giving those phenomena meaning and interpretation. Values are inherent in the selected labels, therefore, assumptions and values inherent in labels must be carefully analyzed. Concepts are continually changing and acquiring new meanings and new attributes (Rodgers & Knafl, 1993). Time, sociopolitical structures, utilization, and perceptions of clients and clinicians contribute to the evaluation, refinement, and mutation of concepts. Concepts are known to be the bricks or blocks upon which the structure of a theory is built. Concepts could be operationalized into variables, which reflect some empirical referents.

Science

Science is a unified body of knowledge about a phenomenon. It is knowledge that is produced through systematic research processes; the answers are considered credible and supported with some shared, agreed upon set of criteria. Science defines the product and the means by which questions are answered with authority. "It is a system of procedures for gathering, verifying, and systematizing information about reality" (Namenwirth, 1990, p. 19) or an aspect of reality, and it is the content that reflects that aspect of reality. Science in a human practice-oriented discipline reflects awareness and consciousness of the student to the politico-cultural values and represents the subjective views of the participants in science making. Nursing science includes the voices of human beings who participate in the scientific processes, as well as the consciousness of the dynamic interplay between science as reflecting reality and influencing reality.

Nursing science includes research, theoretical formulations, and theories that reflect the discipline phenomena. However, the prevailing world view in nursing is that scientists are researchers, whereas theorists are conceptualizers of reality. The dichotomizing of theorists and researchers fails to consider that the aim of research is to generate theory, and that research that is not built on theoretical premises and frameworks tends to answer discreet questions that may not be coherent or have the potential for advancing the knowledge base in a more integrative way.

Metatheory

Metatheory is a theory of theories. The goal of metatheory is to define the types of theories to be generated, ways by which theories are generated and strategies by which theories are evaluated. A metatheorist is equivalent to a methodological researcher who defines and develops designs, addresses issues in the research process, criteria for critique, and strategies for using more appropriate and congruent methodologies. Metatheorists speak about and analyze theories or develop processes for theory development or evaluation, but they do not develop the content of theories. When they do turn to the development of theory content, they are considered theorists, not metatheorists.

Theory Support

Theory support is the process and the product of evaluating theories against a set of criteria and determining their value. Theory support is geared toward establishing the credibility and utility of theories. Theory support includes the appropriateness of describing and explaining nursing phenomena, as well as new insights gained by these descriptions and explanations. Support can be obtained through philosophic analyses, conceptual analyses, existing data, meta-analyses, synthesis of utilization studies, narrative analyses, and analyses of personal journals, as well as through conducting studies that support the utility of the theory and its predictive potential (Meleis, 1995; Silva & Sorrell, 1992).

References

Barnum, B. J. S. (1994). **Nursing theory: Analysis, application and evaluation** (4th ed.). Philadelphia: J. B. Lippincott.

Becher, T., & Kogan, M. (1980). **Processes and structure in higher education.** London: Heinemann.

Bhimer, H. (1969). **Symbolic interactionism: Perspective and method.** Englewood Cliffs, NJ: Prentice -Hall.

Bleier, R. (1990). **Feminist approaches to science.** New York: Pergamon Press.

Kaplan, A. (1964). **The conduct of inquiry: Methodology of behavioral science.** San Francisco: Chandler

Kuhn, T. S. (1977). **The essential tension: Selected studies in scientific tradition and change.** Chicago: University of Chicago Press.

Kuhn, T. S. (1970). **The structure of scientific revolutions** (2nd ed.). Chicago: University of Chicago Press.

Laudan, L. (1981). **A problem-solving approach to scientific progress.** In I. Hacking (Ed.), Scientific revolutions (pp. 144-155). New York: Oxford University Press.

Laudan, L. (1977). **Progress and its problems: Toward a theory of scientific growth.** Berkeley, CA: University of California Press.

Mead, G. H. (1934). **Mind, self, and society.** Chicago: University of Chicago Press.

Meleis, A. I. (1987). Theoretical nursing: Today's challenges, tomorrow's bridges. **Nursing Papers, 5(2),** 49-63.

Meleis, A. I. (1991). **Theoretical nursing: Development and progress** (2nd ed.). Berkeley, CA: University of California Press.

Meleis, A. I. (1995). Theory testing and theory support: Principles, challenges and a sojourn into the future. In B. Neuman (Ed.), **The Neuman systems model** (3rd ed., pp. 447-458). Norwalk, CT: Appleton and Lange.

Merton, R. K. (1973). **The sociology of science.** Chicago: University of Chicago Press.

Namenwirth, M. (1990). Science seen through a feminist prism. In R. Bleier (Ed.), **Feminist approaches to science** (pp. 18-41). New York: Pergamon Press.

Oldnall, A. S. (1995). Nursing as an emerging academic discipline. **Journal of Advanced Nursing, 21,** 605-612.

Parsons, T. (1951). **The social system.** New York: Free Press.

Rodgers, B., & Knafl, K. (1993). **Concept development in nursing: Foundations, techniques and applications.** Philadelphia: W. B. Sanders.

Silva M., & Sorrell, J. (1992). Testing of nursing theory: Critique and philosophical expansion. **Advances in Nursing Science, 14(4),** 12-23.

Toulmin, S. (1972). **Human understanding** (Vol. 1). Oxford: Clarendon Press.

Turner, R. H. (1968). The self conception in social interaction. In C. Gordon & K. J. Gergen (Eds.), **The self in social interaction** (pp. 93-106). New York: Wiley & Sons.

Chapter 6
Philosophy, Theory, and Research in Nursing:
A Linguistic Journey to Nursing Practice
Mary Cipriano Silva

Nursing theory is not a closed book (Levine, 1995).

Nursing theory is not a closed book, and neither is nursing philosophy nor nursing research. Since the emphasis on modern nursing theory that was evident in the 1960s, modern nursing metatheory in the 1970s and early 1980s, and modern philosophy of nursing in the late 1980s and 1990s, nurse theorists and philosophers have grappled with the conceptualizations and linguistic expressions of terms related to philosophy, theory, and research. The purpose of this chapter is to take the reader on a journey—my own personal linguistic journey from 1977 to the present. This journey will reflect the turning pages of an open book, with each page representing my reflections on *key* terminology related to nursing philosophy, theory, and research. The end point is how philosophy, theory, and research inform and empower nursing practice.

Overview of My Linguistic Journey

In 1977, an article of mine was published in *Image*. In reviewing that article, it is clear that I was influenced by logical empiricism but did not totally buy into it. The reason for this was that often my intuition informed me more in "scientific" matters than did my intellect. In that article, I offered three implications for nursing research, which overall I still believe:

1. Ultimately, all nursing theory and research is derived from or leads to philosophy.
2. Philosophic introspection and intuition are legitimate methods of scientific inquiry.
3. Nursing knowledge arrived at by the scientific method too often sacrifices meaningfulness for rigor. (Silva, 1977, pp. 61-63)

In 1984, my journey continued with a coauthored article that appeared in *Advances in Nursing Science* (Silva & Rothbart, 1984). The thrust of that article was that logical empiricism, with its emphasis on logic, deduction, and probable truth was not advancing all of nursing science and the time had come to think about science in a different way. Thus, in that article we focused on historicism, with its emphasis on research traditions, science as process, and a theory's problem-solving effectiveness as evidence of scientific progress.

As I continued to reflect on theoretical and metatheoretical matters in nursing, I noticed a long-standing professional call for the testing of nursing theory. However, few nurse scholars and researchers seemed to understand this concept. My linguistic journey then took me along a path where I examined 62 studies framed by select conceptual models of nursing (Silva, 1986, 1987). In the 1986 article, I formulated seven criteria that, in my mind, would constitute theory testing in nursing. Only 9 of the 62 studies met my criteria. In the 1987 article, I analyzed and critiqued these 62 studies for their use of select nursing conceptual models as a basis for the researches. In 1992, I, along with a colleague, expanded the concept of theory testing to include critical thinking, personal experiences, and application to nursing practice (Silva & Sorrell, 1992).

Finally, I have become fascinated with the increased shift in nursing from quantitative research to qualitative research and the increased shift in society from the knowledge age to the information age. Both of theses shifts represent differing worldviews. Instead of the philosophic emphasis being on how one comes to know (epistemology), the current emphasis is on the nature of reality, meaning, and being (ontology) (Silva, Sorrell, & Sorrell, 1995). Thus, in 1995, my linguistic journey has taken me full circle—back to philosophy, theory, and research.

With this overview of my linguistic journey completed, I will now define *key* terminology related to philosophy of nursing, theory, and research. These definitions have evolved over the course of my journey since 1977 and represent my current thinking. However, the pages of my book remain open.

Linguistics of Philosophy and Philosophy of Nursing

Philosophy and philosophy of nursing are intrinsically intertwined; that is, philosophy of nursing cannot extricate itself from philosophy in the broadest sense. Both are dynamic; both are concerned with wisdom; both are concerned with values; and both strive for abstract universal visions that can be defended through critical powers of the mind but cannot be empirically tested by scientific methods.

There are differences, however, between philosophy and a philosophy of nursing (Kikuchi & Simmons, 1994). Philosophy as used here is a discipline with its own major areas of focus. These areas include, but are not limited to, epistemology, philosophy of science, metaphysics, philosophy of mind, philosophy of language, ethics, social and political philosophy, philosophy of religion, and aesthetics (Earle, 1992).

Regardless of area of focus, philosophy examines all that is known or unknown or all that is explicable or inexplicable in light of first causes. First causes take us or attempt to take us to the essence of things. An example of a first cause question might be, "What is the meaning of life?" Koestenbaum (1968) puts it well:

Philosophy asks the very last questions which the human mind is capable of formulating, and it examines the ultimate foundations in our understanding of man, the world, and their connections. Specifically, philosophy lays bare all implicit assumptions, theories, and methods in any belief whatsoever, and it systematically organizes, structures, and relates all the data and experiences that are available. (p. 21)

In contrast to philosophy, a philosophy of nursing is not a discipline; nursing is. Nursing as used here is a discipline with its own major area(s) of focus. I am basically in agreement with the definition proposed by Newman, Sime, and Corcoran-Perry (1991) that the focus of the discipline of nursing is "the study of caring in the human health experience" (p. 5). Inherent in this vision are the central phenomena and values of *caring, human, health*, and *experience*. Although I believe that these four concepts are necessary to the focus of nursing, I do not believe that they are sufficient.

Now here is where a philosophy of nursing enters. A philosophy of nursing focuses on how nurses raise powerful questions about, seek answers to, and thoughtfully defend their perspectives about the abstract universal visions and values that are *central to nursing*. Nursing focuses on those areas that are central to the discipline of nursing, whereas philosophy focuses on those areas that are central to the discipline of philosophy. A philosophic question that a philosopher might ask is, "What does it mean to be human?" This is a metaphysical or, more precisely, an ontological question. A philosophic question that a nurse might ask is, "What does it mean to be a patient or client?" This is a nursing question with philosophic import. As such, it is linked to philosophy, yet it maintains its loyalty to the discipline of nursing.

Linguistics of Theory and Nursing Theory

Theory
Theory's home base is philosophy, specifically epistemology. Epistemology is that branch of philosophy that deals with "questions of *knowledge* proper, questions of *truth*, and questions of *method*" (Koestenbaum, 1968, p. 20). Epistemology is important because it does not single out any one branch of knowledge to extol but instead examines the essence of *all* knowledge. A part of all knowledge is theory. In keeping with Koestenbaum's definition of epistemology, it follows then that theory involves *knowledge, truth*, and *method*.

How, then, might theory be defined within an epistemological context? Theory is a type of *knowledge* that possesses the possibility of *truth* as determined by one or more *methods* of verification. What is the type of knowledge that is called theory? Philosophers do not agree on the nature and definitions of theoretical phenomena. They do, however, seem to agree that the vast majority of scientific theories contain terminology that cannot be directly observable. These terms are called *theoretical terms*, and the phenomena they refer to are called *theoretical entities*. Furthermore, philosophers deal with the concepts of "incommensurability" and "theory-ladenness" when they discuss theory. The language that a particular theorist or scientist uses in defining and describing his or her theory is said to be "theory-laden" (Earle, 1992, pp. 68, 71).

It follows, then, that no two theories are alike linguistically; this dissonance between and among theories renders them incommensurable. Despite this incommensurability, philosophers believe that communication about the knowledge inherent in various theories is possible because of the vast shared extratheoretical vocabulary that persons of a common culture share (Earle, 1992, pp. 68, 71). In sum, then, at least some philosophers define theory as theoretical entities that can be broad (generic) or particular (theory-laden), that serve some useful purpose for science (e.g., knowledge development) or for a particular science, and that refer to entities that cannot be directly observable but are communicable.

Nursing Theory

Just as philosophers do not agree on the nature of theoretical phenomena, nurse metatheorists, theorists, and nurses do not agree on the nature and definitions of nursing theoretical phenomena. Given that nurses purport different worldviews formed by their cultures, personal experiences, and educational backgrounds, to name a few, it is not surprising that nursing theory is defined in a myriad of ways. I find the variety of definitions interesting, useful, and helpful in moving the discipline forward. This is not to say that a variety of definitions may also foster confusion about nursing theory. But, to me, confusion should be viewed as a positive challenge to critically examine one's own and others' thinking.

How do these preceding thoughts relate to my definition of nursing theory? Since the publication of my first article on theory in 1977, I have seen an evolution in my thinking about nursing theory. My early definitions reflected what I had been taught during my doctoral program—a time when I felt more like a novice than an expert learner in metatheoretical and nursing theory matters. In accord with the stages discussed in Benner's (1984) book, I initially followed the rule bound stage of the novice; that is, I followed what I was taught with little questioning. Inasmuch as logical empiricism dominated the professional literature (not the philosophic literature) at that time, my early definitions of nursing theory had a logical empiricist thrust.

As I progressed on my linguistic theoretical journey, I developed more knowledge and experience in metatheory and in nursing theory. Logical empiricism did not seem to fit my worldview, which was more holistic than reductionistic, more intuitive than empirical, and more creative than objective. Thus, my thoughts about the nature of nursing theory began to change, along with an increasing conviction that how nursing theory was defined was far less important than why nursing theory was important. Today I offer students several definitions of nursing theory and allow them the freedom to select a definition that has meaning for them in research and/or practice. My own definition is as follows:

Nursing theory is an inductively and/or deductively derived collage of coherent, creative, and focused nursing phenomena that frame, give meaning to, and help explain specific and selective aspects of nursing research and practice.

Having put forth this definition, I offer two caveats. First, the definition is dynamic and ever-changing as the philosophic underpinnings of the profession change. Second, the impact of nursing theory—not its definition—takes precedence.

Linguistics of Truth, Method, and Testing of Nursing Theory

As noted previously, theory involves knowledge, truth, and method. Knowledge was addressed in the preceding section; in this section the emphasis is on how truth and method influence theory testing in nursing.

Truth

Philosophers agree that when they address truth, they are talking about what is true as it refers to statements, not true in the expressional sense of a "true" friend. Thus, philosophers focus on what they call propositional truth (Earle, 1992, p. 30). However, how philosophers define propositional truth varies. First, five theories of propositional truth are presented. Next, how these theories have influenced my definition of and methods for testing of nursing theory are discussed.

Earle (1992) presents the most significant theories of propositional truth. First, he notes the disappearance or no-theory theory of truth. It purports that "*p* is true just means that *p*" (Earle, 1992, p. 31). The disappearance theory focuses on the premise that what is, is. For example, "It is snowing" is true just means "It is snowing."

Earle (1992) also asserts the correspondence, the coherence, the pragmatic, and the assertibility theories of truth. The correspondence theory of truth purports that "A statement is true IFF [if and only if] it corresponds with reality" (Earle, 1992, p. 32). The correspondence theory focuses on the premise that beliefs, thoughts, or words must fit real states of affairs, that is, objective facts.

The coherence theory of truth purports that "A statement is true IFF it coheres with all true statements" (Earle, 1992, p. 33). The coherence theory focuses on the premise that consistency and not contradiction exists among any given entities.

The pragmatic theory of truth purports that "A statement, *p*, is true IFF believing that *p* is pragmatic" (Earle, 1992, p. 35). The pragmatic theory focuses on the premise that something is true because a belief in that something is practical, useful, or workable.

The assertibility theory of truth purports that "A statement, *S*, is true IFF *S* is assertible" (Earle, 1992, p. 36). The assertibility theory focuses on the premise that what one asserts is congruent with reality.

In summary, then, each of the preceding theories of propositional truth offers a different definition, focus, and method. Each theory also has its unique strengths and limitations. However, taken together, these theories increase nurses' understanding of what constitutes truth or a lack thereof. Moreover, some understanding of truth is essential for a philosophy of nursing, for the testing of nursing theory through research, and for the application of knowledge to nursing practice.

Method of Testing Nursing Theory

What is meant by testing of nursing theory? How do the preceding theories of truth relate to testing of nursing theory? It seems to me, in a metatheoretical sense, that nurses test nursing theories (or more accurately, aspects of nursing theories) to determine whether they are "true." Empirical nurse researchers tend to focus on the correspondence theory of truth when testing nursing theory. Nurse theoreticians tend to focus on the coherence (deductive theoreticians) and on the pragmatic (inductive theoreticians) theories of truth when testing nursing theory. Nurse clinicians tend to focus on the pragmatic and the assertibility theories of truth when testing nursing theory.

In my 1986 and 1992 articles in *Advances in Nursing Science*, I addressed testing of nursing theory. In 1986, I formulated seven formative evaluation criteria that served as a method for distinguishing testing of nursing theory from other types of evaluative criteria in nursing research:

1. A purpose of the study is to determine the underlying validity of a designated nursing model's assumptions or propositions.
2. The nursing model explicitly is stated as the theoretical framework or one of the theoretical frameworks for the research.
3. The nursing model is discussed in sufficient breadth and depth so that the relationship between the model and the study hypotheses or purposes is clear.
4. The study hypotheses or purposes are deduced clearly from the nursing model's assumptions or propositions.
5. The study hypotheses or purposes are empirically tested in an appropriate manner.
6. As a result of this empirical testing, indirect evidence exists of the validity (or lack thereof) of the designated assumptions or propositions of the model.
7. This evidence is discussed in terms of how it supports, refutes, or explains relevant aspects of the nursing model. (Silva, 1986, p. 4)

These seven criteria were an attempt to elucidate and define what testing of nursing theory meant to me at that time. Then I most likely would have defined testing of nursing theory as a deductive method of verifying through empirical research whether select theory propositions from a given nursing theory supported or refuted the propositions. I do not hold this definition today; I find it too confining.

The impetus for my change of thinking came from within as a colleague and I reflected on what it means to test theory (Silva & Sorrell, 1992). First, we reasoned that scholars in certain disciplines such as philosophy and mathematics do not test theories empirically but nevertheless do test theories. Their method of testing theories is not the scientific research method but rather critical reasoning. By critical reasoning we mean using the highest powers of the mind to analyze, synthesize, and make sense of the phenomena under study. [Although we did not address intuition in the 1992 article, we both now agree that intuition as method is also important in the testing of nursing theory. We agree with Kelly's (1994) definition of intuition as "trusting the everyday whole-knowing of the inner voice" (p. 129).]

Second, we reasoned that shared personal experiences about a common phenomenon constituted a type of theory testing. As we noted in the 1992 article:

> Personal experiences involve direct participation in one or more events that lead to one's own enhanced knowledge, insight, or wisdom, allowing one to verify the "correctness" of those experiences. Personal experiences can be powerful, predictive, and sometimes exclusive types of knowledge, accessible to and verifiable by only those who have experienced them. (Silva & Sorrell, 1992, p. 17)

The method involved here is an inductive process by which each person's seemingly unique personal experience is validated by others with the same seemingly unique personal experience. Perceptions of reality are tested against similar perceptions of reality until a common shared experience is validated.

Third, we reasoned that nursing theory could be tested in practice. In contrast to the testing of nursing theory through the three prior methods where the testing focused on whether what was purported or experienced was indeed so, the testing of nursing theory in practice often uses a different method. This method focuses on problem-solving effectiveness. Laudan (1977) is one proponent of this method. He notes:

> The first and essential acid test for any theory is whether it provides acceptable answers to interesting questions: whether, in other words, it provides satisfactory solutions to important problems. (p. 13)

Nurse clinicians have excellent problem-solving skills, so they are in an ideal position to determine whether important nursing goals have been attained or vexing nursing care problems have been satisfactorily solved. In addition, this method of nursing theory testing intuitively resonates with nurse clinicians, because it is familiar to them and is client centered. Thus, as Reed (1995) notes, "nursing practice [serves as] a metanarrative for knowledge development .... [It] is regarded not only as a place of applying knowledge, but also as a place to generate and test ideas for developing knowledge" (pp. 78-79). I might add that nursing practice is also an excellent place to test the validity of the knowledge that has been generated.

From my thoughts in the preceding section and from my continued journey into the realm of the linguistics of theory testing, I now offer my current definition of testing of nursing theory:

> Testing of nursing theory is a complex deductive-inductive-intuitive process that evolves from an understanding of a philosophy of nursing, of the importance of nursing theory, and of the interrelationships among nursing research, critical reasoning, personal experiences, and nursing practice. Its goals are to verify to the degree possible the truthfulness or the problem-solving effectiveness of nursing theory in clinical or other nursing practice.

Conclusion

In conclusion, my journey has come to an end, but the pages of my book remain open. Because I am a holistic thinker and because I do not like to micromanage linguistic phenomena, I have selected only *key* terms related to nursing theory to define, and I have placed them within philosophic and pragmatic contexts. I have tried to show linguistically how the interrelationships among philosophy, theory, and research in nursing all lead to nursing practice.

Levine (1995) noted that "theory is the poetry of science" (p. 14). I would like to expand that thought. Philosophy-theory-research is the poetry of science. And the poetry takes on powerful new meanings when it is applied in nursing practice.

References

Benner, P. (1984). **From novice to expert: Excellence and power in clinical nursing practice.** Menlo Park, CA: Addison-Wesley.

Earle, W. J. (1992). **Introduction to philosophy.** New York: McGraw-Hill.

Kelly, K.J. (1994). **The nature of intuition among nursing staff development experts: A Heideggerian hermeneutical analysis.** Unpublished doctoral dissertation, George Mason University, Fairfax, VA.

Koestenbaum, P. (1968). **Philosophy: A general introduction.** New York: Van Nostrand Reinhold.

Kikuchi, J. F., & Simmons, H. (Eds.). (1994). **Developing a philosophy of nursing.** Thousand Oaks, CA: Sage.

Laudan, L. (1977). **Progress and its problems: Toward a theory of scientific growth.** Berkeley, CA: University of California Press.

Levine, M. E. (1995). The rhetoric of nursing theory. **Image: Journal of Nursing Scholarship, 27,** 11-14.

Newman, M. A., Sime, A. M., & Corcoran-Perry, S. A. (1991). The focus of the discipline of nursing. **Advances in Nursing Science, 14(1),** 1-6.

Reed, P. G. (1995). A treatise on nursing knowledge development for the 21st century: Beyond postmodernism. **Advances in Nursing Science, 17(3),** 70-84.

Silva, M. C. (1977). Philosophy, science, theory: Interrelationships and implications for nursing research. **Image 9,** 59-63.

Silva, M. C. (1986). Research testing nursing theory: State of the art. **Advances in Nursing Science, 9(1),** 1-11.

Silva, M. C. (1987). Conceptual models of nursing. In J.J. Fitzpatrick & R. L. Taunton (Eds.), **Annual Review of Nursing Research** (Vol. 5, pp. 229-246). New York: Springer.

Silva, M. C., & Rothbart, D. (1984). An analysis of changing trends in philosophies of science on nursing theory development and testing. **Advances in Nursing Science, 6(2),** 1-13.

Silva, M. C., & Sorrell, J. M. (1992). Testing of nursing theory: Critique and philosophical expansion. **Advances in Nursing Science, 14(4),** 12-23.

Silva, M. C., Sorrell, J. M., & Sorrell, C. D. (1995). From Carper's patterns of knowing to ways of being: An ontological philosophical shift in nursing. **Advances in Nursing Science, 18(1),** 1-13.

Chapter 7
Terminology in Theory:
Definitions and Comments
Maeona K. Kramer

Philosophic Orientation

I am pleased to provide a chapter defining theoretical terms for this monograph. I applaud the editors for asking authors to comment on their rationale for choice of definitions. Shared understandings can only help to advance our individual and collective work in nursing science for the benefit of clients. As you read the following definitions and comments, please keep in mind that I do change my mind about things as my understandings and experiences alter. So, what I believe and understand about theory today may not hold for tomorrow. For some entries, there seems to be no reason to comment on why I hold a particular definition. I found myself commenting for those definitions that seem to hold several, often controversial, meanings.

While is difficult to pinpoint epistemological sources for the terminology in this chapter, I recognize that my thinking has been shaped by theoretical positions congruent with my experiences as a nurse, a scholar, and a woman. The publication of Barbara Carper's (1978) work on the Knowing Patterns was highly important for me. Carper's ideas gave voice and legitimacy to some of my own thinking and served as a powerful personal energizer for deconstructing the dogma and challenging the givens surrounding theory in nursing. If I were to name the intellectual traditions that are centrally important shapers of my thought, probably critical feminist and critical social theory would be at the top of the list. These theoretical positions continue to challenge me to undermine our theoretical certainties in the quest for, and questioning of knowledge.

I am well aware of how difficult it is to provide definitions that eliminate instances of illogic between and among meanings. Some definitions will overlap with others, and astute readers will probably find instances of illogic even though I have tried to eliminate them. I invite readers to share their ideas with me in the interest of refining our mutual understandings and ability to communicate them. And, finally, when terms overlap with those contained in *Theory and Nursing* (Chinn & Kramer, 1995), I have often borrowed heavily from that work, providing page references for direct quotes. For some overlapping terms, however, my views may be somewhat different from those set forth in *Theory and Nursing*.

Terminology Defined

Theory

In its broadest sense I regard theory as a partial view or perspective on reality. Theory's partial nature underscores the given that theory, even at its best, can never fully represent reality. This definition of theory is incomplete, however. Theory is also a mediate form of knowledge, meaning that it "goes-between" some forms, or types, of reality and our formal understanding of that reality. The mediate nature of theory means it is represented symbolically and in nursing, usually in language systems. Thus, theory is representational knowledge. Also, the symbolic system that comprises theory must be abstracted in a rigorous and systematic way, further adding to the evolving definition. Rigorous abstraction processes for theory help insure that the partial view of reality it provides is an adequate and trustworthy view.

In *Theory and Nursing* (Chinn & Kramer, 1995), the definition of theory is: "a creative and rigorous structuring of ideas that project a tentative, purposeful and systematic view of phenomena" (p. 71). This definition reflects the view that, in addition to requiring rigor, theorizing is a creative endeavor. What to theorize about, how to derive, structure, and relate concepts or variables, how to represent them definitionally as a way to point users to reality referents, and the assumptions inherent in theory are not universal or standard givens. Because the theoretician will have to choose from among alternatives in carrying out theory development processes, the endeavor is assumed to be creative. Creativity and rigor are not seen as opposites. Rather they co-exist. Including creativity in a definition of theory underscores a hope that theory will move us forward into new ways of thinking about and conceptualizing nursing realities, rather than representing our world in a way that is regressive. The use of tentative in the definition underscores my view that theory is a reflection of the language systems we have available to us as well as our current understandings of reality. As those understandings change and language systems alter, the representational meaning for concepts and assumptions within the theory, indeed for the whole theoretical structure, will change. Thus, theory cannot be anything but tentative. The definition includes the idea that theory is purposeful to call attention to the fact that no theory is neutral. Regardless of whether a purpose is articulated by the theorist, every theory has one. Calling attention to purpose helps underscore the need to attend to the personal and political consequences of theory in nursing.

Meta-theory and Domain/Content Theory

Simply stated, meta-theory is theory about theory within the discipline, whereas domain or content theory is theory about the practice, nature , or direct work related endeavors of a discipline or profession. In nursing, domain theory would be theory about nursing. Meta theory theorizes about the nature of what counts as knowledge (knowledge includes theory), which knowledge structures are important, and how to structure knowledge within the discipline. Domain theory is developed using a particular metatheoretical viewpoint. In differentiating meta-theory from domain theory, concepts within the theory are key. For example, a meta theory would theorize about such things as the nature of concepts important in nursing, types of assumptions nursing should make and their significance, and whether research is the best process for obtaining theory in nursing. A domain theory would include nursing concepts as directed by the metatheory such as "client satisfaction" or "chemotherapy induced nausea." I have found it important to differentiate "theory" into metatheory and domain theory to help with precision in thinking about theory. When asked for references for "nursing theory," for example, questions such as: Do you mean domain theory or metatheory? generally help people broaden their conceptualization of theory and understand the various forms it can take.

Nursing Theory

Nursing theory is content or domain theory containing concepts that reference, or symbolize, ideas pertinent to patient or client care. I do not usually include theory that structures knowledge about the administrative or non-client teaching practices of nursing within the umbrella of nursing theory. Using nursing theory, then, requires access to clients and families. Since it is the nature of the concepts and what they reference that determines whether theory is nursing theory and not the discipline of origin for the theory, nursing theory can be borrowed from other disciplines. Carefully developed domain theory from within the profession, however, is more likely to be "nursing" theory since theoretical processes such as referencing of concepts and choosing assumptions are likely to be more congruent with our practice. Nursing theory developed outside the discipline needs careful scrutiny for appropriateness within the nursing arena.

Empirics/Empirical

In the general sense, I take empirics to mean the doctrine or belief that knowledge derives from experience. This implies that empirically based knowledge does not exist a priori, but flows from a variety of forms of direct and indirect sensory experiences. Empirical theory is formed when information gleaned from sensory experience is structured and organized consistent with credible conceptions of theory. Empirically based theory is also differentiated from other types of theory on the basis of its assessment for credibility. Empirical theory can be assessed for its truth value by an appeal to the senses. If empirical theory is further identified as scientific empirical theory, it implies a derivation utilizing a particular set of research processes—those associated with objectivism. These research processes define the nature of sensory experience that counts as data (more direct experiences), and the rules by which data are observed and quantified. Thus, "scientific" empirical theory is more aligned with traditional methods of science. Less scientific forms of empirical theory are associated with more naturalistic methods of inquiry. In these forms of inquiry, the observational data upon which the theory is based is more indirectly experienced. Thus, I would characterize theory developed out of interview data as empirical theory, but would not term it scientific.

I propose a distinction between empirical theory and scientific empirical theory because I believe that often empirics and science are used synonymously. With the current trend to deconstruct the notion that the only credible knowledge form is scientific theory, interchanging the terms empiricism and science is risky. We stand to lose a lot of valuable nursing knowledge if we begin to generally devalue all empirical knowledge because it is equated with traditional science. Calling attention to the distinction seems important in order to develop additional forms of empirical knowledge which are important to the profession.

Ethical Theory

Ethical theory is theory which addresses moral imperatives—the rights, oughts and shoulds of our practice (ethical nursing theory is assumed) about which there are no single good answers and legitimate disagreements about the best course of action co-exist. Ethical theory can be thought of as either normative or descriptive. Normative ethical theory is systematized using "logical" thought processes and does not require research processes for its derivation. *Normative ethical theory* is like empirical theory in that its concepts derive from sensory experience, but normative ethical theory does not require direct, or even indirect, observation as a basis for structuring and relating concepts that form theory. Rather, concepts can be organized and structured based on long past observations, feelings, and understandings (experiences) within the theorist's memory. Unlike empirical theory the credibility of normative ethical theory is not assessed through reference to valid and reliable sensory data. Rather, it is assessed on the basis of its internal "logic" (rationalism) and the potential and actual results of its use. A "good" ethical theory would produce outcomes that were both just and caring. *Descriptive ethical theory* is a type of empirical theory that systematizes information such as facts or beliefs about the practice of ethical and moral behavior. Theoretical structures that account for what groups of people actually believe or know about ethical challenges such as "physician assisted suicide" would fall within the realm of descriptive ethics. Theoretical structures that account for what people should believe and do about such ethical challenges would constitute normative ethical theory. The distinction between normative and descriptive ethical theory calls attention to the fact that what people describe as beliefs and actions around ethics can be at odds with what they should do, at least by some theoretical accounts.

Grounded Theory

I define grounded theory in a way that is consistent with the writings of Glaser and Strauss (1967), while recognizing that the meaning of the term in nursing has changed to include a variety of inductively derived conceptual structures and theory, providing that induction evolves from research-related processes. Grounded theory is theory that evolves "from the ground" and assumes a recognizable regularity for empirical processes under scrutiny. In its original sense, grounded theory structured information about social processes. Through a variety of field techniques, data are gathered. Using a constant comparative method of analysis, small units of data are generalized into larger wholes (as concepts) which are further generalized and ordered "under" constructs (a relative designation for a higher order concept—one constructed from multiple concepts), that are still further generalized to fit under an umbrella termed a core variable. The process of grounded theorizing includes a return to the literature during the process of data analysis to guide further theoretical sampling, selective sampling based on emerging results, memoing, and an attempt to formalize the theory. In its less purse sense, grounded theory is any inductively developed theory that generally relies on interviewing and observation to obtain data. Personally, I do not feel strongly about either of these definitions of grounded theory. Keeping the conceptualization of grounded theory as proposed by Glaser and Strauss (1967) in mind seems important, however, as it illuminates the significance of grounded theory as an reactionary alternative to grand sociological theories operating at the time it was proposed. For example, Glaser and Strauss's focus on theory formalization is seldom seen as part of the common conception of grounded theory processes, yet understanding that aspect of the process calls attention to historical attempts to render grounded theory as credible as other forms of theory.

Grand Theory

Grand theory is very broad scope theory as determined by examining the purpose, concepts, and definitional components of the theory. Grand theory is a term that is perhaps the closest "opposite" for grounded theory, and was the model for sociological theory which grounded theory opposed. The term grand theory is also often associated with hypothetico-deduction as a method for testing and developing theory. The hypothetico-deductive method of theory building is associated with traditional science and refers to using a structured set of presumed truths (rather than established laws) to deduce relationships/observations for testing. Once observations are made, the deduced relationship is either established or refuted (the context of justification). Attending to grand theory and its historic ties to hypothetico-deduction is an important reminder of the need to be concerned about how grand theories relate to the world of practice—how they were established in the first place (the context of discovery). It also calls attention to the misnomer associated with the phrase "testing theory" because it highlights the fact that such theory testing can only proceed partially.

Macro-Micro Theory

Like grand theory, macro theory is defined as theory that covers a broad range of phenomena. Micro-theory is theory that covers a narrow range of phenomena. These are relative distinctions which I have retained due to their still occasional use in the literature.

Mid-Range Theory

Like macro and micro theory, mid-range theory is a relative distinction in relation to the scope of concepts and purpose within theory. Mid-range theory falls somewhere between micro theory and macro or grand theories. Grounded theories often tend to be within the range of scope of mid-range theories. I think of mid-range theories as having concepts that represent a partial view of nursing practice (such as Mischel's [1988, 1990] uncertainty theory rather than representing the full scope of nursing practice (such as Watson's [1985] caring theory). Mid-range theories in nursing are often more fully research developed and validated than macro or grand theories.

Holistic Theory

Holistic theory reflects the tenets of holism. This means it reflects, through its assumptions, concepts, definitions, structure, relationships, and purposes, that the "whole" which the theory is about is expressed in "parts" that are *both* interrelated and interdependent. Moreover, parts and wholes co-exist simultaneously, that is, any one "part" so designated is at the same time a "whole." This characteristic of holistic theory carries with it an assumption of non-linearity for time and four dimensionality for space. Holistic theory reflects considerations that the whole cannot be understood by an isolated examination of parts, for once parts are isolated the whole no longer exists. A theory tends to be holistic when it does not insist on control as an appropriate outcome for human phenomena. Holistic theories encourage examining parts only in relation to the whole (since the whole determines the parts). I believe that it is important to define holistic theory in a way that respects the tenets of holism as fully as possible since the human organism is holistic in nature. Conceptualizing something called "holistic theory" is somewhat of an oxymoron (since theory by its linearity and language expression cannot really express holism) but still a valuable ideal. Theory that is more consistent with holistic tenets is more valuable to our practice than atomistic theory (defined below) since the theory itself has to acknowledge its limitations in accounting for human behavior. I resist defining holistic theory as simply broad range theory, because one can have broad range theory that does not embody holistic tenets. Macro theory, for example, can be atomistic or holistic.

Atomistic Theory

Atomistic theory assumes that discreet interacting elements comprise a whole. These elements, while interrelated, are not interdependent. Thus, atomistic theory requires an assumption that boundaries exist between and among elements and that if one understands the parts and their interactions, knowledge of the whole accrues. In atomistic theory, a part is a part and a whole is a whole, so any given element could not be part and whole simultaneously. Rather, parts aggregate to form a whole. Atomistic theory is consistent with linear concepts of time and three-dimensional space. In examining atomistic theory, it is permissible to look at the effect of part upon part as a way to gain knowledge of the whole. When applied to the human organism, atomistic theory also assumes the whole is not an emergent that changes and alters with "whole"-"part" interaction, but rather an organism seeking a steady state within an external environment.

Conceptual Framework/Conceptual Model

These refer to a network of concepts, in relationship, that account for broad nursing phenomena. I take the terms conceptual framework and conceptual model to be synonymous. While "model" carries the connotation of physical structure and "framework" the connotation of a language structure, when the modifier "conceptual" is added to either word, the idea that what is modeled or framed are concepts is highlighted, making the terms more or less synonymous. At this point, I am struggling with how to differentiate between conceptual frameworks/models and theory. While I see conceptual models as a type of theory, I do not see all theory as a conceptual models. This is because the terminology of conceptual frameworks/ models is reserved for broad nursing phenomena which not all theory reflects. Another difference between conceptual frameworks/models and theory that is emerging for me, is the extent to which both are actually or potentially grounded in research or other processes of scholarly "validation." At this point, a definition of theory is emerging for me that may reserve the term empirical theory for more "mid-range" formulations that have been derived from research related processes, or that are amenable to validation and testing using empirically based processes. Non-empirical theory (such as normative-ethical theory) in the mid-range, however, is not as easily differentiated from conceptual frameworks. Thus, it seems to me that differentiating between conceptual models/frameworks and theory, if done, requires a conceptualization of theory as "scientific-empirical" in nature, which I am reluctant to do because I want to include broader formulations of theory within my definition of that term.

Paradigm

Paradigm is an overarching "world-view or ideology" (Chinn & Kramer, 1995, p. 76) that organizes ideas, perspectives and systems for knowing about reality. Paradigms determine one's assumptions about reality and, therefore, determine what is important to know, what is a credible way to know about it, and how to represent what is known. Paradigms are ideology in the sense that they determine and limit allegiances to various forms of knowing and knowledge.

Knowing

Knowing is the processes whereby we understand, recognize, feel, sense, act upon and generally experience life. While knowing often tends to be associated with conscious cognitive processes, knowing can reflect a subconscious awareness of events or phenomena we experience. Knowing is ongoing and fluid and a variety of sensory and non-sensory (in the traditional sense) experiences contribute to what we know. Knowing can never be fully expressed to others because it is interactive, fluid, holistic in nature, and ever emerging.

Knowledge

Knowledge is what can be structured and represented to others out of the processes of knowing we experience. Knowing is a process; knowledge is a representation of that knowing which, at best, is partial. Knowledge is often expressed in language. Thus, we usually think about knowledge being written—but knowledge can take other forms such as art, music, and body movement. I believe that it is important to distinguish between knowledge and knowing because we tend to equate knowledge and knowing and assume knowledge in nursing is only structured in form and depends on research or other forms of scholarly inquiry for its existence. Differentiating between knowledge and knowing calls attention to the presumption that knowing is much broader than knowledge, and that there will always be aspects of knowing that we cannot fully represent. Thus, "defining nursing" and "being accountable for our practice" —the rhetoric of what we must do, is going to be an impossible feat in a complete sense, because nursing depends on knowing that cannot be totally accounted for and represented to others.

Practice Theory

I use the term practice in two ways. In the first and broader sense, practice theory includes nursing theory (as defined above) and also would also include theory about the practice of nursing, particularly the functional arenas of nursing that support, but lie outside the context of direct client care. Thus, administrative theory and teaching related theory would fit within the umbrella of practice theory, but would not be considered nursing theory. Used in this broader sense, concepts within practice theory would be in the mid-range and could be referenced fairly directly in practice.

In the second and less broad sense, practice theory refers to the metatheoretical approach of philosophers Dickoff and James (1968) and the resultant theory generated from using that approach. I have found this less broad conceptualization of practice theory to be the most widely held. Usually, when I say "practice theory," people hear "Dickoff and James." Practice theory consistent with the Dickoff and James conceptualization is structured into goal content, prescriptions, and survey list, and their view of practice theory is well explained in their writing. I tend to favor defining practice theory more broadly than that prescribed by Dickoff and James' metatheory. Principally, I think it is important not to see practice theory as existing in opposition to more scientifically grounded metatheory which the Dickoff and James concept tends to encourage. But I do not want to totally disconnect the notion of practice theory from the ideas of Dickoff and James. Their contribution to re-visioning the role of theory in nursing was, and still is, undervalued and underappreciated. To summarize, I favor retaining a notion of practice theory that underscores the essential reason for our discipline's existence that embodies, but is not limited to, the Dickoff and James concept of practice theory.

Praxis Theory

As practice (taken to mean non-revolutionary practice) is beginning to be differentiated from praxis (taken to mean revolutionary practice), I am beginning to define a type of theory that might be termed praxis theory. Since practice theory has been so intimately tied with extant practice, and that practice is highly problematic for a health oriented, holistically grounded profession, it seems important to think about praxis as an important orientation for theory. While the original meaning of practice and praxis were synonymous, praxis is evolving into a term that is associated with revolutionary action that liberates persons "into" critical consciousness and release from oppressive ways of thinking and behaving. Praxis theory goes beyond practice theory to examine and challenge the status quo (e.g. challenge practice theory) with the intent of transforming practice based on a vision congruent with values and ideals. Praxis is grounded in an assumption that social inequities and various oppressions exist. It examines and analyzes the broader contexts which affect nursing practice. Praxis theory would include, for example, theoretical structures that illuminate how ideologies operate to maintain oppressive social conditions for marginalized persons served by nursing. It might also illuminate how those ideologies operate in relation for the profession as a whole. Nursing theory for praxis would suggest ways of being and doing with clients that increase their critical consciousness and liberate them toward increased awareness about available health related choices and the consequences of various courses of action. Since practice theory is criticized on the grounds that it tends to support oppressive practice conditions, defining a form of theory that attempts to undo such inequities seems important.

Critical Theory

Critical theory usually implies critical social theory, which is theory that critiques structures in society that have been constructed to dominate and oppress human potential. The subject matter of critical theory are social structures which seem natural yet create imbalances and inequities in access to social resources. Critical social theory seeks to uncover and deconstruct dichotomies necessary to maintaining oppressive structures. Critical theories stand in opposition to traditional scientific theories. Unlike traditional scientific theories which aim to control human behavior, the aim of critical theories is emancipation and enlightenment. While traditional scientific theories attempt to objectify, critical theories are reflective, and are part of what they are trying to describe. Thus, the "metatheory" of critical social theory and the "domain theory" generated when critical approaches are used tend to merge as the process of critically theorizing proceeds. Scientific theories require empirical confirmation which critical theories do not depend on for validation.

Feminist Theory

In general, feminist theory is theory which structures knowledge about the creation, maintenance, and transcendence of women's oppression. While feminist theory is highly diverse, it various branches are common in two ways. First, all feminist theory shares a common assumption that women, as a class, are oppressed. Second, all branches of feminist theory share the common goal of attempting to account for women's systematic oppression. Feminist theories diverge in their foci and approaches to illuminating the various mechanisms by which women's oppression occurs (e.g., whether oppression stems from unequal property distribution or their childbearing function) and can be transcended. Since various feminist theories account for women's oppression differently, the solutions to the "woman's problem" will vary depending on the theoretical approach. Feminist theory can also include theoretical accounts of women's successful overcoming of oppressions, which is important to acknowledge in its definition.

References

Carper, B.A. (1978). Fundamental patterns of knowing in nurisng. **Advances in Nursing Science, 1**, 13-23.

Chinn, P.L., & Kramer, M.K. (1995). **Theory and nursing: A systematic approach** (4th ed.). St. Louis: Mosby-Year Book.

Dickoff, J., & James, P. (1968). A theories of theories: a position paper. **Nursing Research, 17**, 197-203.

Glaser, B., & Strauss, A. (1967). **The discovery of grounded theory**. Chicago: Aldine.

Mischel, M.H. (1988). Uncertainty in illness, **Image: Journal of Nursing Scholarship, 20**, 225-232.

Mischel, M.H. (1990). Reconceptualization of the uncertainty in illness theory. **Image: Journal of Nursing Scholarship, 22**, 256-262.

Watson, J. (1985). **Nursing: Human science and human care: A theory of nursing**. Norwalk, CT: Appleton-Centruy-Crofts.

Chapter 8
The Language of Nursing Knowledge: Saying What We Mean
Rosemarie Rizzo Parse

"Come, we shall have some fun now!" thought Alice. "I'm glad they've begun asking riddles—I believe I can guess that," she added aloud.
"Do you mean that you think you can find out the answer to it?" said the March Hare. "Exactly so," said Alice.
"Then you should say what you mean," the March Hare went on.
"I do," Alice hastily replied. "At least—at least I mean what I say—that's the same thing, you know."
"Not the same thing a bit!" said the Hatter. "Why, you might just as well say that 'I see what I eat' is the same thing as 'I eat what I see'!" (Carroll, 1960, p. 95)

Philosophic Orientation

Words are symbols of meaning with denotations and connotations. The denotations are explicit definitions or equivalences that signify something directly. The connotations are suggestions derived from non-explicit images evoked by words. The connections of words with the meanings about a notion or idea form a language. Language is an evolutionary patterning of symbols specifying meanings for the moment; it is fluid and ever-changing. All language evolves gradually as generative ideas dawn, shifting the meaning of words and systems of words. The language of science is no exception; thus, my definitions of the language of nursing knowledge are for the moment and will change as new ideas forge different meanings. I created these definitions over time, through concentrated abiding with the knowledge worlds of science, art, and the humanities. These are substantive meanings that reflect synthesized denotations and connotations, and they vary from the definitions used by others in the nursing literature. Many terms referring to nursing theory are used differently by nurse scholars, and it is important to note that these differences reflect a diversity of thought. Meanings in one system of thought vary from those in others; thus, the worldview of the author should be considered when seeking understanding of the meaning of certain words.

Terminology and Definitions

The definitions presented here clarify the meanings of terms that I frequently use. The terms are: *nursing, discipline, worldview, paradigm, phenomenon of concern, science, sciencing, schools of thought, theory, assumption, conceptual framework, theoretical framework,* and *model.*

Nursing is a discipline, the practice of which is a performing art (Parse, 1992, 1995). The performing art is living the disciplinary knowledge.

A discipline may be referred to as a realm, sphere, or domain. It is a branch of knowledge ordered through the theories and methods evolving from more than one worldview of the phenomenon of concern. The parameters of a discipline are always shifting, reflecting the expansion of knowledge.

Worldview is another word for paradigm, which is a philosophic stance about the phenomenon of concern to a discipline (Guba, 1990; Kuhn, 1970; Parse, 1987). Each discipline has more than one paradigm.

A phenomenon of concern is the core focus of a discipline and is stated at a philosophic level of abstraction so as to encompass all manifestations of the phenomenon within the discipline. It may also be called the metaparadigm of the discipline, because it is the reference point for theories and methods from all worldviews. The core focus of nursing, the metaparadigm, is the human-universe-health process (Parse, 1992). The hyphens between the words create a unitary construct incarnating the notion that the study of nursing is the science of the human-universe-health process (Parse, 1992). Consequently, all nursing knowledge is in some way concerned with this phenomenon.

Science is the theoretical explanation of the subject of inquiry and the methodological process of attaining knowledge in a discipline; thus, science is both product and process. Moreover, science is not static but ever-changing and open to the new. The predominant connotation of the term science is that of product. Sciencing, the verbal noun form of the word science, better expresses the meaning of science as process. The term sciencing was introduced by Leslie White (1938) in an effort to foster the notion that science is more than sets of facts specifying absolute truths. I regard sciencing as coming to know through creative conceptualization and formal inquiry. Creative conceptualization is a playful process of reflecting and contemplating phenomena to imaginatively construct ideas. Formal inquiry is the process of coming to know through use of specific research methodologies. Research is the formal process of seeking knowledge and understanding through use of rigorous methodologies. Creative conceptualization and formal inquiry happen within the context of the scholar's worldview or paradigm in general and a knowledge tradition in particular.

Paradigms house the schools of thought within a discipline. Each paradigm contains compatible schools of thought based on general beliefs about the phenomenon of concern. A school of thought, also referred to as a province, is a theoretical point of view held by a community of scholars. Each school of thought is a knowledge tradition that includes a specific ontology (belief system) and congruent methodologies (approaches to research and practice). This means that each school of thought within a paradigm has a theory and consistent methods of inquiry. For example, in nursing there are at least two paradigms or worldviews (the totality and simultaneity) and several schools of thought within each (Parse, 1987). The totality paradigm posits humans as biopsychosocial spiritual organisms adapting to the environment, and health as a state of well-being. The simultaneity paradigm posits humans as unitary beings in mutual process with the environment, and health as a value-laden process (Parse, 1987). The Orem school of thought from the totality paradigm has its own tradition, an ontology (suppositions, presuppositions and three theories), and methodologies (both research and practice). Questions about self-care phenomena are studied within this school of thought, and findings enhance Orem's theories. Parse's school of thought, from the simultaneity paradigm, has its own tradition including an ontology (assumptions, principles, structures), a congruent practice methodology (illuminating meaning, synchronizing rhythms, and mobilizing transcendence through true presence), and a congruent research methodology (dialogical engagement, extraction-synthesis, and heuristic interpretation). Questions about the meaning of experiences of human becoming are studied within this school of thought, and through the findings Parse's theory is enhanced.

Schools of thought are the traditions or streams of meaning cocreated over time through discourse which make up the substantive core knowledge of the discipline. Traditions grow slowly through the discourse arising from creative conceptualization and formal inquiry.

A theory and its assumptions make up the ontology of a tradition. Assumptions are written at a philosophic level of abstraction and articulate fundamental beliefs about the phenomenon of concern to a discipline. A theory is a set of interrelated concepts written at the theoretical level of abstraction describing, explaining, or predicting phenomena, making the assumptions more explicit. A theory provides a lens through which the phenomena of a school of thought within a discipline are viewed. In nursing, a theory with its assumptions sets forth a view of the human-universe-health process through interrelating specific concepts in a unique schema, articulating in abstract language the belief system of a school of thought. For example, in the Human Becoming Theory, the principles are the set of interrelated concepts that make up the theory:

- Structuring meaning multidimensionally is cocreating reality through the languaging of valuing and imaging.
- Cocreating rhythmical patterns of relating is living the paradoxical unity of revealing-concealing and enabling-limiting while connecting-separating.
- Cotranscending with the possibles is powering unique ways of originating in the process of transforming. (Parse, 1981, p. 41)

These principles, which are based on congruent assumptions, make up a unique schema articulating a specific belief system about nursing's metaparadigm construct, the human-universe-health process.

A conceptual framework (conceptual system) is a structure of ideas written at the same level of abstraction formulating a blueprint for something. It is more general in nature than a theoretical framework, a configuration of interrelated concepts written at a high level of abstraction. For example, the conceptual framework for the Human Becoming Theory is made up of three major concepts written at the same level of abstraction: meaning, rhythmicity, and cotranscendence. An example of a theoretical framework or structure derived from the Human Becoming Theory is "imaging is the connecting-separating of originating."

Model is another word that is frequently used to mean different things in the nursing literature. I regard a model as something worthy of imitation. A model may appear in different forms. It is a replica, an image or a likeness that represents something and may also be called a schema or a structure. A model may be a figure drawn to show the connections of ideas, or it may be expressed in digital terms, or may even be a plaster cast of something. To avoid confusion, I do not use the term model in describing aspects of nursing knowledge.

Figure 1 depicts the words of nursing knowledge described in this chapter. All of these aspects of knowledge are ever-changing, flowing through, with, and against each other. There is no direct line from which all knowledge arises; the seed may grow out of any aspect to join the flow of the stream of knowing.

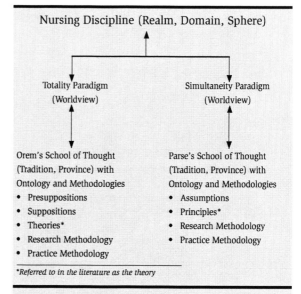

Figure 1. Example of nursing knowledge flow.

Conclusion

The language of nursing knowledge is complex and often confusing because scholars use the same words to express different meanings. These meanings arise from different worldviews, representing diversity of thought within the discipline. Perhaps such diversity contributes to the richness of the discipline of nursing. The words of nursing knowledge are really the meanings, the synthetic notions articulated by the authors of the words. They should be used carefully and in the appropriate context. "You should say what you mean," so that when tracing a stream of knowing through its discourse, a tradition can readily come to light with its basic beliefs clearly in view.

References

Carroll, L. (1960). **The annotated Alice: Alice's adventures in wonderland and through the looking glass**. New York: World Publishing.

Guba, E. (Ed.). (1990). **The paradigm dialog**. Newbury Park, NJ: Sage.

Kuhn, T. S. (1970). **The structure of scientific revolutions**. Chicago: University of Chicago Press.

Parse, R. R. (1981). **Man-living-health: A theory of nursing**. New York: Wiley.

Parse, R. R. (1987). **Nursing science: Major paradigms, theories and critiques**. Philadelphia: Saunders.

Parse, R. R. (1992). Human becoming: Parse's theory of nursing. **Nursing Science Quarterly, 5**, 35-42.

Parse, R. R. (1995). **Illuminations: The human becoming theory in practice and research**. New York: National League for Nursing Press.

White, L. (1938). Science is sciencing. **Philosophy of Science, 5(4)**, 369-389.

Chapter 9
Déjà Vu, Parroting, Buy-Ins, and an Opening

Patricia L. Munhall

The Mission

Could it be true, I ask myself? That after 25 years of theory building in nursing and the development of nursing knowledge, I receive the following request:

> The purpose of [this] monograph is to present several short essays dealing with the specific terminology various nurse scholars use for nursing knowledge and the underlying philosophic and/or pragmatic rationale for the terminology. If you accept this invitation, your chapter should identify the terms you use for nursing theory and metatheory, the definitions of those terms and your philosophic and/or pragmatic rationale for those terminology.

"If you accept this invitation," certainly is reminiscent of Mission Impossible, for those readers in my circa. And déjà vu is another response. Seeking the operational definition, as understanding and knowing, was and I suppose still is, a highly regarded activity in the search for making the intelligible, comprehensible. However, etymologizing or searching for the meaning of words, as though there is universal meaning, or even clear meaning, has long since eluded scholars of knowledge structure and sometimes may even serve as a distraction to more important matters of experiencing "being" in this world. Rather than avoid the invitation to "definition," I would prefer to approach such a task as one of philosophic discourse and "reconstruct" the preoccupation with what I think is often non-contextual epistemology.

I have long since argued against spending undue time on these matters, time lost for substantive inquiry. Suffice it to say that this is the way something is defined, for this purpose, for whatever, in this particular context according to this particular person, who often is the author of a required textbook. Students are undoubtedly influenced by the text that is chosen, in the subtle and not so subtle value statements communicated either within the text, or by the professor.

As an educator, and one of those who choose and suggest books for students, I am keenly aware of this critical step in the educational process. So to proceed with my narrative, "What do I actually do?" or "How do I use these terms" will be directly answered. I have students read *On the Weakness of Language in the Human Sciences* by Gerald Burns(1987) and also some of Heidegger's literature on "covered-up-ness" and appearances and concealments. Assumptions are also critical to these discussions. I go in the back door, so that we can explore the meaning of words in the philosophical, political and practical ways in which they appear within context. What freedom or limitations are inherent in the terminology, is an essential aspect of understanding the power of definitions.

Structural definitions are static and not responsive to the dynamic nature of the universe. With 25 years of bonding with one another (nurse professors and students) through these epistemological discourses, one might postulate that it is indeed time to move on. It seems as though we have an endless capacity to feud over the minutiae of structure instead of turning to substance. Many nurse scholars have abandoned this quest for perfect clarity in the structure of the discipline of nursing and instead have embraced a post-modern perspective where the ideas of contingency, multiplicity and polyvocality are recognized. In so doing, there is the recognition of antithetical theories, which seems like a good thing inasmuch as there are a variety of individuals in the world, a variety of perceptions, and a variety of meanings.

Also it still provides a way of bonding because these differences yield to healthy discourses as well, and to discovery. Time to become unstuck, and understand that uncertainty and ambiguity are part of this mystery that will continue to defy a holding down and a wrestling to squeeze out a static structural model of some sort.

The Emotional Attachment to Words

This way of searching for meaning of words or phrases acknowledges that time, place, and different perspectives will influence the way in which they are used. Individual assumptions, biases, and experiential history also are contributing factors to why words, such as "domains, phenomena of concern, conceptual models, conceptual frameworks, grand theories, paradigms, research programs, and integrative science," remain steeped in ambiguity. Cannot the very discourse about this language include the recognition that individuals cognitively take in some type of "what this means" and can repeat it for the sake of a qualifying examination, and yet the word still remains meaningless without comprehension of the political and philosophic implications of the words? Clearly, understanding and "restatability" are two quite different realms.

Considering this period of time, however, when many of us grew up in nursing, there is a strong emotional attachment to these words and ideas, and we continue to perpetuate the same language. It provides a sure footing, security and keeps the same debate going. Now it is passed to the next generation. This bond of structure was at one time needed but I think we are emotionally mature enough to raise the level of discourse to one that is more meaningful and substantive. And probably much more philosophic, political, and sociological.

Parroting

In nursing, especially in graduate education, there often seems to be an indoctrination process. A value on "restatability," a joining with a theorist, and a "buy-in" to a particular paradigm all are evident. Frequently, the student has little choice but to "parrot" the prevailing norms to progress.

We might be quick to recognize this as being antithetical to the liberating purpose of education but we would be naive to think that in most institutions of higher learning it is otherwise. In fact, the most frequent admonition to graduate students is to do what is expected, do what your committee wants, and when you graduate you can do your own "thing."

Please allow me to digress, by way of a personal example of how specificity in terminology can be a method of indoctrination, and a way of stifling creativity, as well as wondering about alternative ways of conceptualizing. Let me tell you about my own experience in graduate education, which I think many graduate students and colleagues will recognize readily.

Déjà Vu

I'll call this story Déjà Vu.The year was circa 1968. I entered graduate school and "theory" was in vogue. Knowing the difference between a theoretical framework and a conceptual framework was critical. Arguing whether various theorists actually had a theory or not was done as though life itself depended on such a determination. I was in a school where the "buy-in" was not a choice but a requirement. Skip ahead six years. Now I enter another school for a doctorate, choosing this school in particular because I thought "buy-in's" were not required, and I could experience freedom of exploration. Advance now to dissertation time. Although it was true that a student did not have to join with a particular theorist, so to speak, she/he had to join with a particular paradigm, which at the time was logical positivism. (In this instance, "paradigm" meant, "This is how one does research. This is the one true way." In addition, there was no plural sense to the word, such as paradigms.) That was painful for me because I did not dwell so much in that world as I did in another, which had far greater meaning to me. But I followed the pragmatic advice of "doing the expected" and "don't create waves."

As I write this, I am thinking that in graduate education, one could cogently argue that for knowledge to advance, students should be encouraged to do the unexpected and create many waves. If that were the case, this book would not be needed. Apparently, we are still embroiled in the search for specifics in terminology, which should be guideposts or maps and quite flexible as the terrain changes. The implicit value system that accompanies this terminology also is quite distressing.

There seems to be a ranking order of superiority, which is not grounded so much in what is important but what is more dominant or considered more scientific. Perhaps even what faculty know best. Professors, including myself, are often invested in some way in this process of assigning greater value to one theory or paradigm than another. This, I think, is inevitable, yet the danger would be in using one's own preferred theorist or method in the indoctrination of students. However, when a student becomes excited by a specific theory for reasons that make particular sense for meaningful practice and research, in a way that she or he constructed with a great amount of reflection, than that can be wonderful. When a "something" that can become a passion for one's work is found, the process of "work" is perceived almost as a transcendental experience. The critical point, though, is that "something" comes from the spirit of the individual and not as a "requirement."

Take, for example, all that terminology, and say, "What difference does it make? There are more significant subjects to explore. Let us move on with real questions about the world, its people, the conditions of our society, and the problems that need brain power and brain energy to solve." If the terminology questions, which are 25 years old, are still being ruminated upon, perhaps there *are* no specific or satisfying answers, so how long should we massage them? Let us instead redirect our energy to life-like questions, not abstractions and epistemyzing about structure instead of, for example, hunger, poverty, homelessness, racism, intolerance, people's physical and emotional pain, fear, anxiety, and loss of hope.

Again I have digressed. Back to the story. Now we move ahead several more years to about 1983, and I'm at a faculty meeting, where the discussion is about faculty development workshops. A suggestion is offered and is very popular as a topic. That topic is the differences between a conceptual framework and a theoretical framework, what is really a theory and what is not, what kinds of theories are there, and what is scientific and what is not. Obviously, great value was, and still is, placed on terminology and the structural definition of the terms. There was a great search for certainty. That is when we liked doing concept clarification. Those were the days; everything could be defined, if you just labored long enough.

That part of our theoretical history brought patterns of adaptation, categories of defenses, developmental stages for both living and dying, differential diagnosis definitions, and communication theory, as well as family and organization theories. Although they served as compasses and a possible explanation for some phenomena, we come to know that the contingencies of being human reflect the proverbial belief that "all knowledge is tentative." Though "knowledge may be power," outdated knowledge becomes obsolescent and weak.

So we readily accept, for instance, that theory in physics that is one year old has probably changed, and that family theory that is 10 years old no longer serves its purpose due to the changing demographics and fabric of what a family is as we enter the next century. Revisionist theory is essential to encompass societal changes and social and political contingencies. Critical theory is essential to philosophically analyze the power structure inherent in advancing specific theories. Who is to gain? Who will keep the power and class structure? That is how I discuss theory, paradigms, and metaparadigms. I use the most accepted and easily understood ways of conceptualizing the terminology and than move on.

I have to admit, though, that the discussions of the 1970s and 1980s did, and still do, drive me to distraction. I guess that if you have read this far, my frustration is readily apparent. I once wrote an article, in verse, that demonstrates for the sake of this story how I would reply to the questions raised in this monograph. So now we advance to the year 1986. These verses in their entirety appeared in *Advances in Nursing Science* (Munhall, 1986), in an article entitled, "Methodological Issues in Nursing Research: Beyond a Wax Apple." A few excerpts continue the quest to answer how I particularly conceptualize terminology.

Answering These Questions in 1986

This is into the article a bit:

wax apples
analogue models, systems, stages, symmetry
tasteless, dry, but perfect in stability
and lifelessness
definitions, like wax apples
limit possibilities (Munhall, 1986, p.2)

Thus, in this brief essay, it would be contrary to my belief system to provide definitions for terms. In teaching, I give examples of what the contemporary thinking is concerning terminology and encourage students to understand the experience of thinking about these kinds of things. I ask them, "What does it mean?" A "thinking through" of various paradigms, including logical positivism, biological materialism, existentialism, and phenomenology, is more important, as is a going "inside" them, an exploration of what they are and what they are not. And from a post-modern perspective, does one need to rank order or choose?

But I have gotten ahead of myself here with that question; back to 1986. It is hard to believe that this is still relevant, at least for the questions posed, and that in itself is quite revealing, considering the length of time that has elapsed. Here is some more:

We come and go
Are we pre-paradigm or metaparadigm?
or no paradigm and a
research tradition
Are we qualitative or quantitative
Are we empiricists, historicists or past it
all? (Munhall, 1986, p.2)
And about "isms:"
so I think its OK to have an "ism"
so long as I don't equate it to "truth" (Munhall, 1986, p. 3)

In nursing in 1986, antithetical images or theories were not considered useful or even possible for a science. There was a concerted search for the "right" answer. Of course, "right" answers only give us a partial picture of what might be right in one particular context. The same with a theory, which is time and context bound. Our theories are class and culture bound. So it behooves us to be open to multiple perspectives and multiple ways of being and embracing of differences. Spending 25 years on this kind of concept clarification without acknowledging the perspectives from which such analysis arises is perhaps why the questions do not go away.

Assumptions

Probably the most important term, and that term was not mentioned in the prospectus for this monograph, is "assumption." I suppose it is part of my own journey that I arrive at a place and think about the "truths" we take for granted, that undergird knowledge, i.e., assumptions, and believe that is what we should be discussing. What a leap to think that our, for the most part middle-class, assumptions from a very select group of people, are representative of a population. It seems to me that it would be helpful to understand that perhaps there is no best way, there is no one best outcome, there is no one definition. On that, back to 1986.

> We seem though (understandably considering the anxiety)
> to want rules and corresponding rules
> We seem to search for truth
> Impregnable citadels
> Where the hopes, fears and loves
> of human beings (self care agents) are
> distracting (Munhall, 1986, p.5)

Since 1986, I have practiced not being distracted by these hopes, fears, and loves of human beings. I have also tried to examine my own middle class worldview and the audacity that perhaps I should "instruct" others to think like me or like others I may come across in the literature. When I engage in "teaching," a privilege that I highly respect, I have become wide-awake to my own assumptions, biases, and preconceptions. Surely there is inclusion of terminology, but as guideposts and as different ways of thinking about reality.

A Buy-In

There is also discussion about what happens with a "buy-in" to a theory or paradigm. There is discussion about choosing a way of thinking about reality. What is excluded from this perception? Who is excluded from this perception? Do we have the ethical prerogative to impose these perceptions on others, in particular students and patients? Many of our theories are constructs of inclusion and exclusion. They are prescriptive for a specific socioeconomic class.

Alas, that is not the purpose of this piece. Critiquing theory is another topic, one that I would dare say is essentially more vital to a discipline than our endless capacity to be diverted over the use of terminology.

Meaning

In the process of education, educators need to make important choices. All subject matter cannot be taught, hence decisions have to be made. Theory courses and the explication of the structure of the discipline are, however, staples in graduate education. The selection of paradigms, theories, and the research methods that are advanced often is biased. Restatability is often the outcome. Analysis is permissible as long as, in the end, the student realizes the correct answer.

Students are "taught" about metaparadigms, domains of knowledge, concepts, etc.—the "banking" concept of teaching. Pour information into this empty vessel, indoctrinate, and than withdraw the information to ascertain if the balance is correct (Belenky, 1986). In contrast, the "construction of knowledge" concept of learning is to assist students to find what is inside themselves and their experiences and construct knowledge based on contingency, interpretation, and meaning. This approach is enormously growth producing for students as they talk and explore their own language. They learn from listening to one another how misdirected a prescription from theory might be. They create in the new day, in the new context.

The philosophy of phenomenology now guides my educational place in the world. The search for meaning becomes pivotal. However, lest I be accused of indoctrination, doing and practicing in a phenomenological way is always a choice. So when asked how I use specific terminology, I would say I use it to explore the meaning that the words have in the context of understanding human experience (Munhall, 1994). Searching for meaning is one of many possible ways of being in the world. Some philosophies and their compatible theories may focus on the search for patterns, or relationships, or attaining goals, or self-care. This does not necessarily exclude one from another. Perspectives and searches can be multiple and, indeed, could be richer for the inclusions.

Multi-Mind

This is the magnitude of "multi-mind," a twenty-first century concept of postmodernism. As we move into the next century, trying as hard as we did for control and prediction in the last century, we acknowledge the flux, the unpredictable, the uncertainty, the ambiguity, and the mystery. This mystery resides in each of us and cannot, I believe, be reduced to categories, stages, formulas, and structural definitions.

In Coming to an Opening

The opening is the ongoing group of nurses who continue to move with time; nurse theorists and/or philosophers who say contingency, power, culture, means revisioning theory. The time is now postmodern. We have learned much from the modern time, the good, the forgettable. Looking at history, we were off base with many of our predictions. Our enemies are now our allies, and one could say they may be enemies in another time once again. We could not have predicted AIDS in populations that suffer from discrimination or moral judgement. We did not predict the information highway, and that "cyberspace" would be a common concept. Yet we still have cancer, and mastectomies, and colostomies, and mental illness, and childhood accidents, and malnutrition, and violence at home and in society. Our opening to these experiences will come with a fresh way of perceiving them. That has always been the way. We might once again call it a paradigm shift but all new ages were a shift in providing new visions. Whatever, let us provide the opening. Struggling with structural definitions is too static, yet it has helped us realize that experience cannot be captured in a definition.

Resolves

I suggest that we no longer talk about crossroads, critical points in our theory development, even the next century, which is arbitrary. Although I know that I did that very thing in this chapter, I suggest that we move on this continuum in an evolving manner, as a moving stream, following the course of the stream, wherever it takes us. I suggest that we be alert to contingencies, alert to individual perceptions, alert to individual and cultural meanings, alert to our own class values and from this, respectful of differences. And I truly believe the only way to get from here to there is to resolve to LISTEN. Listen, without comment; listen, with encouragement; listen, and we will learn from master story tellers, individuals who have experienced things we may not have. Let us LISTEN to our students, patients, and significant others, to come to know the mysteries, and values, and desires of those we care about. Let us think through and about and not define or categorize. Individuals, both listener and speaker, grow in this way in understanding and knowing that, which is truly constructed knowledge.

One last quote from 1986:
Struggle to the surface from didacticism
to the freedom
of possibilities
of uncategorizing
the colors for time, space, & being (Munhall, 1986, p.1)

References

Burns, G. (1987). On the weakness of language in the human sciences. In J. S. Nelson, A. Megill, & D. N. McCloskey (Eds.), **The rhetoric of the human sciences**. Madison, WI: University of Wisconsin Press.

Belenky, M. F. (1986). **Women's ways of knowing**. New York: Basic Books.

Munhall, P. (1986). Methodological issues in nursing research: Beyond a wax apple. **Advances in Nursing Science, 8(3)**, 1-5.

Munhall, P. (1994). **Revisioning phenomenology: Nursing and health science research**. New York: National League for Nursing Press.

Epilogue

Imogene M. King
Jacqueline Fawcett

As one reads the previous nine chapters, it is difficult not to be impressed with the authors' individual and collective dynamic openness as they share their approaches to knowledge development and the intellectual effort they have expended on behalf of the advancement of the discipline of nursing. Each author has expressed her ideas from a personal background of knowledge and experience as well as from a particular philosophic viewpoint. The diversity of viewpoints, terminology, and definitions reflects the dynamic openness of the discipline of nursing as a whole. Clearly, no single perspective dominates. Consequently, all nurses benefit from the openness of our discipline to multiple perspectives.

Philosophic Orientations

The authors have explained their progression from initial ideas about theory and metatheory, along with their underlying philosophic orientations, to their current thoughts about the nature of knowledge in nursing. Collectively, the nine chapter authors agree that knowledge development for nursing is based on each person's philosophic orientation. The following summary of each author's underlying philosophic orientation highlights the diversity of approaches to thinking about nursing theory and metatheory.

Diversity of Philosophic Orientations

Fawcett has adopted an empiricist orientation. Her version of empiricism is rooted in the postpositivistic position that all knowledge is developed within a conceptual socio-historical perspective, and that all observations are made within a particular frame of reference.

Fitzpatrick's definition of theory is rooted in the philosophic orientation of symbolic logic. Moreover, Fitzpatrick acknowledged the influence of Kuhn's description of scientific revolutions through a process of theory testing on her view of theory and terminology.

Silva related her philosophic journey from logical empiricism to historicism, with emphasis on research traditions. Furthermore, she explained her shift from a philosophic emphasis on epistemology to ontology, with its emphasis on the nature of reality, meaning, and being.

King indicated that her philosophic orientation is rooted in general system theory, which guides the study of organized complexity as whole systems. She pointed out that general system theory provides a holistic approach to studying nursing as an open system, with a focus on the complex interrelationships of social phenomena in natural environments.

Kim noted that her perspective of critical realism is a reconciliation of epistemological realism and emancipatory epistemology. Critical realism, according to Kim, leads to a view of nursing knowledge that is both evolutionary and critical. Kim indicated that she believes that an integrative and synthesizing framework for nursing epistemology needs to be developed.

Kramer identified critical feminism and critical social theory as her underlying philosophic orientation. Meleis has also adopted a feminist perspective, which she indicated provides a platform for relocating definitions and theoretical goals within time and socio-cultural and political contexts. In addition, Meleis acknowledged the influence of symbolic interactionism on her thinking about theory.

Parse discussed words as symbols of meaning with denotations and connotations that form a language. She regards language as fluid and changing and an evolutionary patterning of symbols specifying meaning. Parse noted that a discipline is a branch of knowledge that evolves from more than one worldview of the phenomena of concern.

Munhall has adopted what might be considered an anarchistic philosophic orientation. Indeed, she pointed out that the selection of terms and their definitions are most likely dependent on the momentary context.

Terminology and Definitions

Each chapter author cited the influence of a particular philosophic orientation on preferred terminology and definitions. Systematic examination of the content of the nine chapters, however, revealed little evidence of generalizable linkages between philosophic orientation, terminology, and definitions. For example, both Kramer and Meleis cited the influence of feminism on their thinking but offered somewhat different lists of terms and defined the same terms in different ways.

The explicit articulation of the nine chapter authors' viewpoints and definitions brings clarity, if not consistency, to the terms found in our literature. A definition is no more or less than an agreement to use a word or phrase in a specific way. The diversity of terms used by the nine chapter authors, as well as the various definitions for the same terms, is evident in the glossary at the end of this monograph.

Examination of the various definitions given by the chapter authors to the same terms reveals some agreement about the basic meaning of a term, with differences at a more specific level. For example, Fawcett, Fitzpatrick, King, Meleis, and Parse all agree that theories contain concepts. Each, however, ascribes further, more specific meaning to the term theory.

Levels of Abstraction

Many of the chapter authors pointed out that there are levels of abstraction in nursing knowledge. For example, both Fawcett and Fitzpatrick regard a conceptual model as a high level of abstraction. Moreover, although Fawcett and Kramer used different terms, they agree that theories can be at different levels of abstraction. In particular, Fawcett used the terms grand theory and middle-range theory, whereas Kramer used the terms macro theory and micro theory, as well as the term, mid-range theory.

Future Directions in the Language of Theory and Metatheory

All nine chapter authors agree that scientific knowledge development is an essential responsibility of the discipline. Most also agree that nursing knowledge development is essential for the survival and advancement of the discipline. No specific formula for knowledge development has, however, emerged. In fact, a specific formula would contradict the openness and diversity of the guiding philosophies and terminology that are evident in this monograph.

Some of the chapter authors maintained that the time has come in the discipline of nursing to move beyond discussions of terminology to the development of substantive knowledge. Munhall, for example, commented that "structural definitions...are not responsive to the dynamic nature of the universe," and that "it is indeed time to move on" from epistemological discourse. Furthermore, Meleis noted that "all of the terms have been used interchangeably...that using them interchangeably is inconsequential, [and that] a more productive use of the intellectual and theoretical capabilities of nurse scholars is to debate the substantive issues in the discipline."

Although we agree that nurse scholars should focus on the substance of nursing knowledge, we maintain that an understanding of the language undergirding that substance is crucial. We hope that this monograph will enhance nurses' understanding of the language of nursing theory and metatheory and encourage them to move beyond language to substance. We believe that the openness and diversity of philosophic orientations and terminology that are evident in this monograph can serve as a catalyst for nurses who wish to continue the development of nursing knowledge.

International Implications

International interest in and contributions to nursing theory have been evident throughout the history of modern nursing. International interest in dialogue about nursing metatheory has been especially evident in the past decade, with an increasing number of conferences in several countries and the translation of many books about nursing metatheory into several languages, as well as the international efforts to standardize nursing language for diagnoses, interventions, and outcomes.

We hope that this monograph will serve as a stimulus to nurses worldwide to consider the cross-cultural applicability of the versions of the language of nursing theory and metatheory given by the nine chapter authors. Furthermore, we hope that this monograph will stimulate nurses throughout the world to develop still other versions of nursing theory and metatheory and to continue to contribute to the substance of nursing knowledge.

Glossary

Terminology and Definitions Used by Selected Nurse Scholars

Assumption	Written at a philosophical level of abstraction; articulates fundamental beliefs about the phenomenon of concern to a discipline (Parse)
	A truth that is taken for granted, that undergirds knowledge (Munhall)
	A statement that is taken for granted and accepted, a premise upon which concepts are developed, theories evolve, and research is conducted; a statement considered to have support for high probability of truth; a statement that reflects values, beliefs and/or goals related to a concept, theory, discipline, or nursing action (Meleis)
Atomistic Theory	Assumes that discreet interacting elements comprise a whole; these elements, while interrelated, are not interdependent; requires an assumption that boundaries exist between and among elements and that if one understands the parts and their interactions, knowledge of the whole accrues (Kramer)
Concept	An abstract idea that gives meaning to one's perceptions, permits generalizations, and tends to be stored in one's memory for recall and use in new and different situations (King)
	A linguistic label given to things, events, ideas, and other realities we perceive and think about; a symbolic statement describing a phenomenon or a class of phenomena (Kim)
	An abstract, mental image of a phenomenon with a label that distinguishes it from other phenomena or classes of phenomena; reflects sense observations, inferences, intuitive leaps, and a systematic representation of phenomena (Meleis)
Conceptual Framework	A general perspective of organizing and classifying concepts into a relevant structure (Kim)
	A structure of ideas written at the same level of abstraction formulating a blueprint for something; also called a conceptual system (Parse)
	A mental or physical image of a structure that evolves from a theory or from the integration of a number of theories in some unique way to generate new questions or to view new relationships; also called a model (Meleis)
Conceptual Model	A set of abstract and general concepts and the propositions that integrate those concepts into a meaningful configuration; synonymous with conceptual framework, conceptual system, paradigm, and disciplinary matrix; more abstract than a theory (Fawcett)
	A network of concepts, in relationship, that accounts for broad nursing phenomena; synonymous with conceptual framework (Kramer)
	Constitutes a level of nursing theory [metatheory level] (Fitzpatrick)
Conceptual System	A set of concepts that are defined and linked by broad generalizations constructed by an individual for a purpose (King)

Critical Theory	Usually implies critical social theory which is theory that critiques structures in society that have been constructed to dominate and oppress human potential (Kramer)
Discipline	A realm, sphere, or domain; a branch of knowledge ordered through the theories and methods evolving from more than one worldview of the phenomenon of concern (Parse)
	Provides a unique way of considering the phenomena that are of interest to its members (Meleis)
Domain	Composed of related items for scientific investigation, constituting a unified subject matter that poses important problem(s) for scientific investigation and having the quality of readiness in a scientific sense to deal with the problem the subject matter presents (Kim)
	The crux of a discipline; the territory that shapes both its theoretical and practical boundaries (Meleis)
Domain of Nursing	The domain of nursing assumes person-environment transactions; the domain focus is helping individuals, families, and communities maintain health, which indicates that nursing is a goal seeking system (King)
Domain or Content Theory	Theory about the practice, nature, or direct work related endeavors of a discipline or profession (Kramer)
Empirical Indicators	The very specific and concrete real world proxies for middle-range theory concepts; the actual instruments, experimental conditions, and research procedures that are used to observe or measure the concepts of a middle-range theory (Fawcett)
Empirical Theory	Formed when information gleaned from sensory experience is structured and organized consistent with credible conceptions of theory (Kramer)
Empirics	The doctrine or belief that knowledge derives from experience (Kramer)
Ethical Theory	Theory that addresses moral imperatives—the rights, oughts and shoulds of our practice (ethical nursing theory is assumed) about which there are no single good answers and legitimate disagreements about the best course of action co-exist (Kramer) *Normative ethical theory* is systematized using "logical" thought processes and does not require research processes for its derivation (Kramer) *Descriptive ethical theory* is a type of empirical theory that systematizes information such as facts or beliefs about the practice of ethical and moral behavior (Kramer)
Feminist Theory	Theory that structures knowledge about the creation, maintenance, and transcendence of women's oppression (Kramer)
Grand Theory	Made up of rather abstract and general concepts and propositions that cannot be generated or tested empirically; developed through thoughtful and insightful appraisal of existing ideas or creative intellectual leaps beyond existing knowledge (Fawcett)
	Very broad scope theory as determined by examining the purpose, concepts, and definitional components of the theory (Kramer)
Grounded Theory	Theory that evolves "from the ground" and assumes a recognizable regularity for empirical processes under scrutiny (Kramer)

Holistic Theory	Reflects the tenets of holism, i.e., reflects, through its assumptions, concepts, definitions, structure, relationships, and purposes, that the "whole" which the theory is about is expressed in "parts" that are *both* interrelated and interdependent; parts and wholes co-exist simultaneously, that is, any one "part" so designated is at the same time a "whole" (Kramer)
Knowing	The processes whereby we understand, recognize, feel, sense, act upon and generally experience life (Kramer)
Knowledge	What can be structured and represented to others out of the processes of knowing that we experience (Kramer)
Macro Theory	Theory that covers a broad range of phenomena (Kramer)
Metaparadigm	The global concepts that identify the phenomena of interest to a discipline and the global propositions that state the relationships among those phenomena (Fawcett)
	An analytical framework for a discipline which specifies the guidelines, principles, and procedures with which the phenomena of concern for the discipline are delineated and articulated (Kim)
	The core focus of a discipline, stated at a philosophical level of abstraction so as to encompass all manifestations of the phenomena within the discipline; also referred to as the phenomenon of concern (Parse)
Metatheory	Theory about theory within the discipline (Kramer)
	A theory of theories (Meleis)
	A higher level of theory that could include conceptual models (Fitzpatrick)
Micro Theory	Theory that covers a narrow range of phenomena (Kramer)
Mid-Range Theory	Having concepts that represent a partial view of nursing practice (Kramer)
Middle-Range Theory	Made up of concepts and propositions that are empirically measurable (Fawcett)
	A set of relational statements from which testable hypotheses can be derived (Fitzpatrick)
Model	In science, someone's conceptualization of phenomena, invented for a specific purpose; suggests theories which correlate patterns in observable data; organizes a large quantity of data in a very few concepts (King)
	Something worthy of imitation that may appear in different forms; a replica, an image or a likeness that represents something; may also be called a schema or a structure (Parse)
Nursing	A discipline, the practice of which is a performing art; the performing art is living the disciplinary knowledge (Parse)
	A discipline that includes the content and processes related to the roles that nurses play, such as teacher, administrator, clinician, consultant, researcher, and theoretician, which constitute knowledge communities with a sense of collectivizing; the theories developed to describe, explain, prescribe, or predict the nature of the phenomena with which members of the discipline deal; and schools of research traditions organized to answer the discipline's problems (Meleis)

Nursing Theory	An inductively and/or deductively derived collage of coherent, creative, and focused nursing phenomena that frame, give meaning to, and help explain specific and selective aspects of nursing research and practice (Silva)
Paradigm	A specific scientific tradition in terms of (a) major form(s) of explanation/ heuristic espoused, (b) the perspective with which essential phenomena of concern to a discipline are conceptualized, and (c) the specific commitment to scientific method(s) for knowledge development (Kim)
	An overarching worldview or ideology that organizes ideas, perspectives and systems for knowing about reality; determines one's assumptions about reality and, therefore, determines what is important to know, what is a credible way to know about it, and how to represent what is known (Kramer)
	A philosophical stance about the phenomenon of concern to a discipline; also called a worldview (Parse)
	A shared framework and a shared view held by members of a discipline about the discipline; also called a "disciplinary matrix" or a school of thought (Meleis)
Phenomenon	Designates an aspect of reality existing as a pre-linguistic entity and adopting a linguistic meaning upon human perception, recognition, and experience; all aspects of reality in this sense represent either separate, multiple phenomena or a single phenomenon (Kim)
	A thing, event, or situation that exists in reality and reflects an aspect of reality that is colored by the perception of the view of that reality (Meleis)
Philosophy	A statement of beliefs and values; more specifically, a statement about what people assume to be true in relation to the phenomena of interest to a discipline and what they believe regarding the development of knowledge about those phenomena; also called a worldview (Fawcett)
	A discipline with its own major areas of focus; includes but not limited to epistemology, philosophy of science, metaphysics, philosophy of mind, philosophy of language, ethics, social and political philosophy, philosophy of religion, and aesthetics (Silva)
	Encompasses the values, norms, and beliefs that influence the context of theories and research and the processes utilized in developing them (Meleis)
Philosophy of Nursing	Focuses on how nurses raise powerful questions about, seek answers to, and thoughtfully defend their perspectives about the abstract universal visions and values that are central to nursing (Silva)
	Nurses' orientation to life, their practice, the moral dilemmas they encounter, and the meanings they ascribe to events (Meleis)
Practice Theory	(1) Includes theory about the practice, nature, or direct work-related endeavors of nursing and also theory about the practice of nursing, particularly the functional arenas of nursing that support, but lie outside the context of direct client care; (2) The metatheoretical approach of philosophers Dickoff and James and the resultant theory generated from using that approach (Kramer)
Praxis Theory	Goes beyond practice theory to examine and challenge the status quo (e.g., challenge practice theory) with the intent of transforming practice based on a vision congruent with values and ideals (Kramer)

Research	An organized, systematic, and formal process to solve specific problems or answer specific questions resulting in new knowledge or new relationships among phenomena in a discipline (King)
	The formal process of seeking knowledge and understanding through use of rigorous methodologies (Parse)
Science	To know (King)
	The theoretical explanation of the subject of inquiry and the methodological process of attaining knowledge in a discipline; both product and process (Parse)
	A unified body of knowledge about a phenomenon that is produced through systematic research processes; the answers are considered credible and supported with some shared, agreed upon set of criteria; defines the product and the means by which questions are answered with authority (Meleis)
Sciencing	The verbal noun form of the word science; better expresses the meaning of science as process; coming to know through creative conceptualization and formal inquiry (Parse)
School of Thought	A theoretical point of view held by a community of scholars; each school of thought is a knowledge tradition that includes a specific ontology (belief system) and congruent methodologies (approaches to research and practice); also referred to as a province (Parse)
	A paradigm (Meleis)
Scientific Empirical Theory	Implies a derivation utilizing a set of research processes associated with objectivism (Kramer)
Scientific Knowledge	Results from use of scientific methods in studying natural phenomena (King)
Theoretical Entities	The phenomena referred to by theoretical terms (Silva)
Theoretical Framework	A general perspective of a logically coherent integration of theoretical positions regarding a set of concepts, which becomes the basis for developing a system of related theories (Kim)
	A configuration of interrelated concepts written at a high level of abstraction (Parse)
Theoretical Terms	Terms contained in scientific theories that cannot be directly observable (Silva)
Theoretical Thinking	Components include the processes of analysis of situations, events, and actions that include reflection, connection with other ideas, interpretation, generating meaning, abstracting, comparing, contrasting, and/or utilizing theories to explain situations or guide actions; strategies are to reduce, synthesize, and/or analyze the components; the goals are to integrate into more coherent wholes, develop a more coherent view, and create some order related to ideas where none may have existed and/or where pre-existing wholes are not as illuminating as new proposed integrated wholes (Meleis)

Theory	Made up of relatively specific and concrete concepts and propositions that purport to account for or organize some phenomenon (Fawcett)
	A set of interrelated concepts, based on assumptions, woven together through a set of propositional statements; used to symbolically describe reality; and that reflect an interpretation of reality (Fitzpatrick)
	A set of theoretical statements that provides an understanding and explanation about a class or classes of phenomena (Kim)
	A set of interrelated concepts, definitions, and propositions that present a systematic view of essential elements in a field of inquiry by specifying relations among variables (King)
	A partial view or perspective on reality; a creative and rigorous structuring of ideas that project a tentative, purposeful and systematic view of phenomena (Kramer)
	A mental image of a coherent view of a phenomenon and/or its relationship to other phenomena; an abstract representation of a reality formulated to answer some significant questions; an organized, coherent, and systematic articulation of a set of statements related to significant questions in a discipline that is communicated in a meaningful whole; made up of concepts, descriptive statements, prepositions, and a narrative explanation (Meleis)
	A set of interrelated concepts written at the theoretical level of abstraction describing, explaining, or predicting phenomena (Parse)
	A type of knowledge that possesses the possibility of truth as determined by one or more methods of verification (Silva)
Theory Support	The process and the product of evaluating theories against a set of criteria and determining their value (Meleis)